ESSENTIALS OF
PHARMACOLOGY

ESSENTIALS OF
PHARMACOLOGY

By

D.K. Basu Ph.D,

Professor of Pharmacology and former Principal
A.R. College of Pharmacy, Sardar Patel University, Gujrat.
Former Visiting Professor, Military Medical College, Iraq.

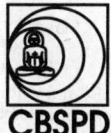

CBSPD

CBS Publishers & Distributors Pvt Ltd

New Delhi • Bengaluru • Chennai • Kochi • Kolkata • Lucknow• Mumbai
Hyderabad • Jharkhand • Nagpur • Patna • Pune • Uttarakhand

Essentials of Pharmacology

ISBN: 978-81-239-1150-2

Copyright © Publisher

First Edition: 1995

Reprint : 2000, 2004, 2005, 2006, 2008, 2009, 2012, 2014, 2017, 2018, 2019, 2020, 2024 **2025**

Published by Satish Kumar Jain and Produced by Varun Jain for

CBS Publishers & Distributors Pvt Ltd

4819/XI Prahlad Street, 24 Ansari Road, Daryaganj, New Delhi 110 002, India.4819/XI Prahlad Street, 24 Ansari Road, Daryaganj, New Delhi 110 002, India.

Ph: 23289259, 23266861   Website: www.cbspd.com
                                               e-mail: delhi@cbspd.com

Corporate Office: 204 FIE, Industrial Area, Patparganj, Delhi 110 092

Ph: 011-4934 4934   Fax: 011-4934 4935   e-mail: publishing@cbspd.com;
                                                                        publicity@cbspd.com

Branches

- **Bengaluru:** Seema House 2975, 17th Cross, K.R. Road, Banasankari 2nd Stage, Bengaluru 560 070, Karnataka
  Ph: +91-80-26771678/79   Fax: +91-80-26771680   e-mail: bangalore@cbspd.com
- **Chennai:** 7, Subbaraya Street, Shenoy Nagar, Chennai 600 030, Tamil Nadu, India
  Ph: +91-44-26680620/26681266   Fax: +91-44-42032115   e-mail: chennai@cbspd.com
- **Kochi:** 42/1325, 1326, Power House Road, Opp KSEB, Power House, Ernakulam 682 018, Kochi, Kerala, India
  Ph: +91-484-4059061-65, 67   Fax: +91-484-4059065   e-mail: kochi@cbspd.com
- **Kolkata:** 147, Hind Ceramics Compound, 1st Floor, Nilgunj Road, Belghoria, Kolkata-700056, West Bengal, India
  Ph: +033-25633055, 033-25633056   e-mail: kolkata@cbspd.com
- **Lucknow:** Basement, Khushnuma Complex, 7 Meerabai Marg (Behind Jawahar Bhawan), Lucknow-226001, UP, India
  Ph: +91-522-4000032   e-mail: tiwari.lucknow@cbspd.com
- **Mumbai:** PWD Shed, Gala no 25/26, Ramchandra Bhatt Marg, Next to JJ Hospital Gate no. 2, Opp. Union Bank of India Noorbaug, Mumbai-400009, Maharashtra, India
  Ph: 022-66661880/89   e-mail: mumbai@cbspd.com

Representatives

- **Hyderabad**   0-9885175004   - **Jharkhand**   0-9811541605   - **Nagpur**   0-8692091830
- **Patna**   0-9334159340   - **Pune**   0-9664372571   - **Uttarakhand**   0-9716462459

Printed at: SRK Graphics, Shahdara, Delhi, India

PREFACE

"Essentials of Pharmacology" has been outlined and designed according to the curriculum of undergraduate studies. The contents of the book are believed to have adequate information for the undergraduate students of Pharmacy and medicine.

The main objective is to present the major text of Pharmacology in an easily retrievable form for use as a ready reference. The format has been selected in order to condense available drug information to just the essentials. Subject matter has been given an upto date coverage and emphasis has been placed on all pharmacological data of therapeutically important old and new drugs.

Important aspects of clinical usefulness and explanations of mechanisms of drug action that are essential for understanding fundamental concepts of pharmacology have been dealt in a manner that would server the student's purpose. Drug interactions, adverse reactions and toxic effects have been incorporated appropriately with almost all drugs.

With deep appreciation I thank Mr. Satish Kumar Jain and Vinod Kumar Jain of CBS Publications for their interest and help in making possible the publication of this book.

I thank Mr. Sunil Dhir of Super Computers for his best efforts in Laser typesetting of this book.

D.K. Basu

CONTENTS

1

FUNDAMENTAL CONCEPTS

Pharmacology is a multidisciplinary study of drugs. It is primarily related to the physiological and biochemical aspects of drug action in relation to its chemical structure. This includes the studies of the absorption, distribution, metabolism and elimination of drugs. Since drugs can produce harmful effects on human beings even in very small amounts administered for the mitigation and cure of diseases, pharmacology also covers acute and chronic toxicity studies.

The qualitative and quantitative drug effect depends on the rate of absorption, distribution and excretion of the drug from the body. This aspect of drug action is referred as pharmacokinetics. The studies of biochemical and physiological mechanism of action and relationship between drug effect with its chemical structure are covered under the term pharmacodynamics.

A drug produces its effect as an ultimate consequence of physico-chemical interactions between the drug and a functionally important site known as receptor. Effects of a drug are produced only when it is present in proper concentration at this receptor site. This site can be present inside or on the surface of the cell.

Many hormones, neurotransmitters and other factors act as extracellular signals to bind first to receptors at the cell membrane surface. The receptor is then activated and binds to a drug in a manner which is not yet understood at the molecular level. However, the pharmacological consequences of this activation are well known and is termed as receptor oriented drug effect.

1.1. ROUTES OF DRUG ADMINISTRATION

Drugs require administration through a specific route to produce a desired effect.

The routes of drug administration can be :

    (i) Enteral

    (ii) Parenteral

    (iii) Inhalation aerosol

    (iv) Topical applications.

1.1.1 Enteral

The enteral routes of administration are oral, sublingual and rectal. For administration through these routes drugs are either in solid dosage form e.g. tablets, capsules or liquid oral preparations e.g. suspension, syrups etc. Oral route is the safest and delivers the medicament slowly into the blood circulation; hence rapid increase of blood concentration is avoided. However, in case of solid dosage forms, the rate of drug absorption is dependent upon its rate of dissolution in the stomach and intestinal fluids. Commonly tablets require administration at definite intervals to produce a sustained drug effect. Therefore, a number of pharmaceutical preparations have been designed as controlled release or sustained release solid dosage forms which result in slow uniform absorption of drug over a long period. Such preparations have an advantage of reduction of frequency of administration.

However, oral drug absorption from solid dosage forms may be irregular because of variation in gastrointestinal pH; gastric emptying and intestinal motility.

Sublingual Route of Administration : Some drugs get extensively metabolized by the liver enzymes. Such drugs if given by the sublingual route can cut off the first pass metabolism, as the venous circulation from the mouth goes to the superior vena cava directly.

Rectal route of administration : This route of administration is useful for unconscious patients and also if there is persistant vomiting. Drugs are administered as suppositories. The drug is made into a solid dosage form in a theobroma oil base which melts at body termperature to release the medicament.

Rectal administration may also produce irregular drug absorption and can cause local irritation.

The disadvantages of enteral administration are :
1. Rate of drug absorption is variable.
2. Irritation of gastric mucosal surface.
3. Some drugs can be subjected to extensive hepatic metabolism. Hence the concentration in blood is affected which in turn reduces the efficacy.

1.1.2. Parenteral

Parenteral routes of drug administration are :
(a) Intravenous
(b) Intramuscular
(c) Subcutaneous
(d) Intraperitoneal
(e) Intrathecal i.e., through the spinal subarachnoid space
(f) Transdermal.

All these routes give a rapid response but due to rapid drug absorption there can be more untoward effects of a given drug. A parenteral dosage form is an injection of a sterile solution of a particular drug. All injections must comply with the specific tests for sterility and other pharmacopoeial requirements.

Injections can produce local irritation at the site of administration.

1.1.3. Aerosol and Inhalation

Volatile drugs like general anaesthetics are administered by inhalation. They produce very rapid action as they are absorbed from the mucous membrane of the respiratory tract.

In addition some drugs can be dispersed as fine droplets as in the case of *aerosol* and inhaler. This also gives a very quick effect.

1.1.4. Topical Applications

These dosage forms are meant for the skin and eyes, e.g. ointments, lotions etc. They produce little systemic absorption.

Ophthalmic ointments and solutions are used for local effect on the eye. However, there can be systemic absorption through the nasolacrimal canal and can cause undesirable side effects. All eye preparations, given as *eye drops*, should be isotonic with lacrimal fluid.

Ocular insert has been developed as a new ophthalmic drug delivery system for prolonged duration of action. They provide low amounts of medicament in a continuous manner and very little drug is lost through nasolacrimal drainage and thus produce minimum side effects in comparison to eye drops.

When a drug is administered in a particular amount the effect produced depends upon dosage and concentration in blood. Concentration in plasma determines its concentration at the site of action which is responsible for the intensity of the effect.

Bioavailability : It is the relative rate at which an administered drug reaches the general circulation. This is of significance if the drug is given orally. The factors influencing bioavailability are :

1. Solubility of the drug in the stomach
2. Food habits.
3. Formulation of the dosage form.

Bioequivalence is the term used for comparable bioavailability between related preparations of drugs.

Therapeutic equivalence stands for comparable clinical effectiveness between drugs.

1.2. DRUG ABSORPTION AND TRANSPORT

Therapeutic effect of a drug depends on its absorption and transport to the active site. To reach the active site the drug has to cross several cell membrance barriers. This is achieved by either of the following processes.

(a) Passive diffusion
(b) Carrier mediated diffusion
(c) Active transport and endocytosis.

Most drugs penetrate cells in an unionized form. Factors that influence this passive diffusion process are :

(I) Molecular size
(II) Lipid water partition coefficient.

Partition coefficient plays an important part because the cell membrane is a bimolecular lipid layer, so the lipid water distribution coefficient and the concentration gradient determine the process of *passive diffusion*. In the diffusion process the drug molecule crosses the lipid membrane and quantity absorbed is related to the molecular size in an uncharged form (unionized). Greater the lipid water partition coefficient, the greater is the drug flux. Since the molecule crosses the lipid membrane in an unchanged form the distribution of the drug is a function of pka of the drug molecule and pH of the surrounding medium.

This can be expressed as

$$Pka = pH + \log \frac{\text{concentration of unionized drug}}{\text{concentration of ionized drug}}$$

The drug can be either a weak acid or a weak base and therefore pH of the medium affects the absorption and excretion of any passively diffused drug. From these considerations it can be explained that aspirin and other weak acidic drugs are best absorbed from the stomach because in the acidic surroundings the drug remains in maximum unionized state. On the other hand basic drugs are best absorbed in the small intestine which has a higher pH that keeps the basic drug in the maximum unionized form.

Another important influence of pH is in the process of drug reabsorption that occurs in the kidney. Since the pH of the urine is acidic a weakly acidic drug can be extensively reabsorbed into the body from the urine. Conversely if the urine is made alkaline the excretion of the acidic drug can be increased and alternatively by making the urine acidic, basic drugs can be excreted rapidly. This process is used in case of acute drug poisoning for the rapid removal of drug from the body.

Passive transport and carrier mediated drug diffusion : Some polar and non polar drug molecules of low molecular weight can diffuse through cell membranes suggesting the existence of channels or pores in the cell membrene. This process of passive transport occurs following the process of filtration.

The capillaries of some vascular beds like that of kidney may have larger pores which permit the passage of large molecules.

Carrier mediated drug diffusion is more specific for particular types of chemical structures of drugs. In this process movement across the tissue membrane is facilitated by macromolecules.

Active Transport : The features that distinguish active transport from passive diffusion process are that in active transport metabolic energy is generated by the enzyme known as Na +-K+ Atpase which transports drug molecules against a concentration gradient.

Drug transport can also occur by a minor process known as *endocytosis.*

In this process certain drug molecules are transported into the tissue cells by a vacuolar apparatus that are present in some cells.

1.3. DISTRIBUTION AND EXCRETION OF DRUGS

Some of the drugs after reaching the circulatory system can bind reversibly and non specifically to the plasma proteins viz. albumin or globulin. As this is a reversible process there is an equilibrium between the bound and free drug. Only the free drug can produce the pharmacological effect and is metabolized and eliminated.

The distribution of a particular drug depends on the blood flow in that region. This factor has important consequences for certain groups of drugs e.g. distribution of barbiturates in the CNS.

Besides this the body has some anatomical barriers which do not allow the free passage of all types of drugs in all areas e.g. blood brain barrier and placental barrier. This implies that all drugs are not readily accessible to the the brain or fetus. Some drugs get trapped in fatty tissues. Eventually the drug which is in free state produces its effect and is then excreted in unchanged form or in metabolized form.

Most drugs are excreted by the kidney. Excretion of drugs or their metabolites occur through the urine, involving glomerular filtration, active tubular secretion and passive tubular reabsorption processes that occur during urine formation. For drugs that are metabolized by the liver, the biliary tract and the feces can be the excretory route. Some drugs and their metabolites are also eliminated in sweat, saliva, breast milk and in the expired air.

1.4. METABOLISM OF DRUGS

The liver is the major site of metabolism for many drugs. The other organs involved are lungs and kidneys. Many factors affect drug metabolism. Chemical properties such as molecular weight and degree of ionization, together with the route of administration play an important part in drug metabolism. For example by the oral route of administration extensive hepatic metabolism (first pass effect) can result with many drugs.

The other factors can be dosage, diet, age, genetic and disease state like renal failure, liver dysfunction and cardiac failure. In renal failure there is slower removal of a drug and therefore administration of the usual dose produces accumulation of the drug which can give rise to toxicity. In kidney failure the renal clearance of drugs excreted through kidney is predictable but it is not possible to predict hepatic metabolism of drugs in liver dysfunction. Therefore, in hepatitis changes may range from impaired to increased drug clearance. In cardiac failure the perfusion of the kidney and liver may also be impaired and can affect drug clearance by these organs directly or indirectly. So in congestive heart failure or hemorrhagic shock the response to the usual dose of many drugs may be excessive and may require modification.

Biochemical reactions involved in drug metabolism are:

   I Oxidation

  II Reduction

 III Hydrolysis

 IV Conjugation.

I **Oxidation :** can be microsomal or non-microsomal.

Microsomal oxidation takes place in a collection of membrane associated enzymes located in the smooth endoplasmic reticulum of many cells, especially in the liver. The enzymes involved are cytochrome P450 mixed function oxygenase and P 450 reductase.

Drugs can inhibit or activate these enzymes.

Non microsomal oxidation : Oxidative enzymes are found in the cytosol or mitochondrial cells such as alcohol dehydrogenase and aldehyde dehydrogenase which are responsible for the metabolism of ethyl alcohol. Similarly, xanthine oxidase, tyrosine hydroxylase and monoamine oxidase are the other examples of non microsomal oxidative enzymes that act on xanthine group of drugs, catecholamines and serotonin respectively.

II **Reduction :** Can be also microsomal or non microsomal. Drugs that have nitro or azide group are subjected to reduction.

III **Hydrolysis :** The enzymes are hydrolases, which act on ester group. For example non specific esterases metabolise acetylcholine, succinylcholine, and procaine like drugs. The other enzymes belonging to the same group are peptidases, phosphatases, and amidases. They metabolize procainamide and nicotinamide like drugs.

IV **Conjugation :** Metabolism of non polar drugs involves coupling of drugs and their metabolites with an endogenous substrate that can be excreted as soluble substances. The substrates are inorganic sulphate or glucuronide. The conjugated drugs are inactive and excreted in urine or bile. Drugs having phenolic, alcoholic, or carboxylic acid group are subjected to conjugation.

Metabolism of drugs can be related to genetic factors. Individuals may differ in the rate of disposition of drugs like isoniazide, hydralazine, procainamide etc. that are metabolized by acetylation.

1.5. TIME COURSE OF DRUG ABSORPTION, DISTRIBUTION AND ELIMINATION (PHARMACOKINETICS).

To produce a specific effect a drug must be present in required concentration at the site of action. In order to be present at the required site of action it must be absorbed from the depot where it has been introduced and be transported to the site through the plasma water of the body. In pharmacokinotics we study about the time course of drug action which may be determined from the rates of drug absorption, distribution and elimination. Therefore the three most important parameters of pharmacokinetics are : bioavailability, clearance and volume of distribution. Bioavailability in its simplest form means the fraction of drug absorbed as such into the systemic circulation. This fraction varies according to the route of administration.

When a drug is administered intravenously the entire dose can be said to be absorbed whereas for drugs that are administered orally, a constant fraction of the dose is absorbed at a constant rate. Information regarding rate of absorption or bioavailability can be obtained by determination of the blood level of the drug at constant interval of time.

Rate of drug absorption : Most drugs are administered by the oral or subcutaneous route or intramuscular injections as drug solution and the absorption follows first order kinetics, i.e. a contstant fraction of the total dose present is absorbed in each equal interval of time. On intravenous administration 100% of the drug is absorbed at one time and is said to follow zero order kinetics.

As the total amount of drug diminishes from the depot the rate of absorption also decreases proportionately. The time course of absorption can be described in terms of the absorption half time, which is the time when drug content of the depot gets reduced to half its initial value.

Elimination : For most drugs elimination from the blood follows exponential or first order kinetics. It has been observed that the decline in the plasma level is almost linear on semilogrithmic coordinates. Therefore elimination half life $(t_{1/2})$ denotes the time at which half the quantity of the drug that was administered is removed from the body.

Distribution of a drug in body tissues : The absorption and elimination kinetics of a drug determines the distribution of the drug in the body tissues. The distribution kinetics of a drug can be based on either of the following model systems where the body is considered as :

(a) One compartment model.

(b) Two compartment model

(c) Multi compartment model.

One compartment model is the simplest and commonly used model for pharmacokinetic calculations.

In this system the distribution of the drug is assumed to be uniform and occurs rapidly in comparison to absorption and elimination. In such a hypothetical situation the body requires an initial (loading) dose and subsequent maintenance doses of the drug to achieve optimal effect. This depends on the kinetics of drug elimination and distribution. However, in practice it has been observed that after intravenous administration almost all of the drug can be accounted in the plasma compartment as shown by high initial plasma level. Ultimately the drug goes into the extra vascular compartment and the period during which this process occurs is known as the distribution phase.

After distribution has proceeded to a point where the concentration of drug in plasma is in equilibrium with that in the tissue outside the vascular compartment the drug starts showing its pharmacological effects.

The drug level in the plasma and body tissues subsequently falls because now it is eliminated from the body. In one compartment model the apparent volume distribution (V_d) can be quantitatively expressed by measuring the plasma level of the drug.

$$V_d = \frac{\text{Total quantity of the drug in body}}{\text{Concentration of drug in blood}}$$

In *two compartment model* we assume that there is a central compartment that refers to the plasma and a peripheral compartment including the extracellular space. In the *multiple compartment model* for accounting the volume distribution a number of factors are involved such as drug storage in the body depots, extensive metabolism and different mechanisms of elimination. In practise estimation of V_d is redundant because drugs do not display ideal behaviour.

Effect of repeated dose administration : On repeated administration of a drug accumulation in the body tissue occurs if the time interval between doses is less than four elimination half time. Total body stores of the drug increases exponentially to a plateau, which is called *steady state concentration*. This is a function of dose, time interval and elimination half life. For drugs administered orally at the half time of elimination the average body store is about I.5 times of the amount administered.

However with I.V. administration after four elimination half life we get 10% of the desired steady state values.

1.6. DOSE-RESPONSE RELATIONSHIP

It has been observed that drugs that produce similar qualitative pharmacological effects can have very different levels of efficacy.

Efficacy is usually more important for clinical considerations than potency.

In order to understand the significance of the terms efficacy and potency we resort to the determination of dose response relationship in a suitable experimental setup.

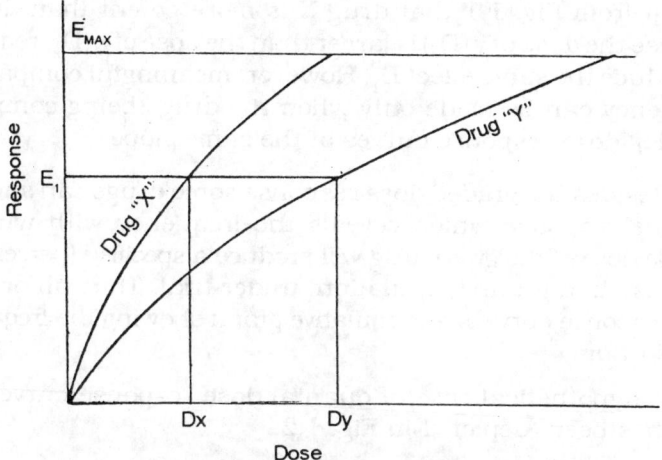

Fig. 1.1 : Graded Dose-Response Curves for two Hypothetical Drugs X and Y. E_{max} = Maximum effect; Dx, Dy = Amount (Dose) of drug x and y respectively required to produce the same effect E_1

The *dose response relationship* can either be a graded dose response or quantal dose response (all or none response) Measurement of the graded dose effect can be carried out on an isolated animal tissue such as frog rectus muscles, guinea pig ileum or rabbit duodenum. The tissue is suspended in an organ bath with suitable attachment that can keep the tissue alive for a considerable period when perfused with an appropriate physiological solution. The isolated tissue is then subjected to a quantitative graded increase in exposure to the drug at definite time interval and for a definite period of contact in the organ bath. The effect of the drug on the tissue can be recorded with a suitable device. As the isolated living tissue is exposed to a drug a pharmacological response is obtained in the form of contraction or relaxation of the tissue tone which can be measured. If this quantised form of effect is plotted against increment in dose of the drug a hyperbolic curve will be obtained. This has been illustrated in Fig. 1.1 where graded dose-response curves for two hypothetical drugs X and Y have been plotted.

Efficacy of these hypothetical drugs can be determined from a comparative measure of potency of two different doses of the drugs that are needed to produce the same effect. It is evident from Fig. 1.1 that drug X is more potent than drug Y because the dose of y (D_y) is larger than the dose of x (D_x) required to produce the same effect E_1. However, meaningful comparison of potency can be made only when the drugs being compared have log dose response curves of the same slope.

Besides the graded dose response some drugs can show all or none response which reveals the frequency with which a specific dose of the given drug will produce a specified (percentage) response in a group (population) under trial. Thus all or none dose response curve is a cumulative graph showing the frequency distribution.

A hypothetical case of quantal dose response curve for a drug has been depicted in Fig. 1.2.

Frequency distribution curve is obtained by plotting the number of subjects (animals or patients) responding against the minimum dose needed to produce the response.

Log dose response curve is constructed for getting a comparison of potency which is independent of efficacy. Simultaneously we obtain an idea of dissociation constant for the drug receptor complex (K_D) which the therapeutic agent forms at the target site to show a pharmacological effect. We also get an estimate of ED $_{50}$ that is the minimum dose showing an effect which is 50% of the maximum effect. In other words ED_{50} is a measure of drug potency. To draw a log dose response curve, log dose is plotted on the X axis (abscissa) and the effect of the drug on the Y axis (ordinate) as represented in Fig. 1.3.

From the graphic representation (Fig.103) we can obtain ED_{50} of two hypothetical drugs A and B where drug A is more potent than drug B. Efficacy is indicated by the height of the log dose response curve. In this case the drug B is less eficacious than A because Emax of the two drugs are quite different. Most drugs combine reversibly with the active site (receptor). If we represent quntatively the drug as 'D' and the receptor as "R"

A graphic representation of frequency distribution curve for a hypothetical drug.

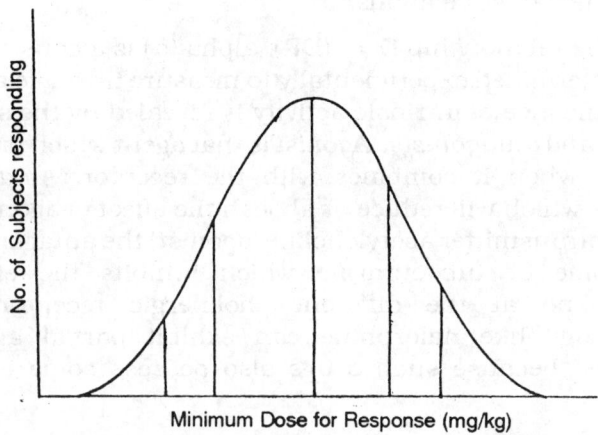

Fig. 1.2 : Curve showing a quantal response (No. of subjects) to a drug against the minimum dose needed to produce the response.

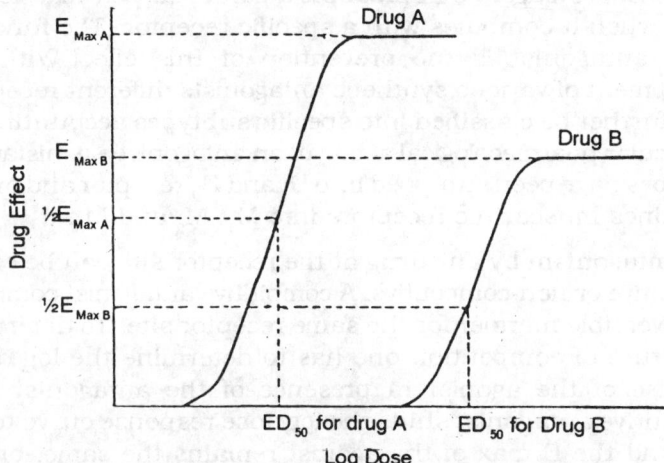

Fig. 1.3 : Log dose-response curve for two hypothetical drugs A and B. E_{MAX} = Maximum effect, ED_{50} = Smallest dose showing an effect that is 50% of E_{MAX}.

then the equation can be represented as $(D) + (R \rightleftharpoons (DR)$; the same can also be represented in terms of quantative expression $E = \alpha(DR)$ where E is a function of the quantity of the drug receptor complex. Magnitude of E always depends on the amount of DR.

So once all the receptors are saturated or occupied by the drug we obtain the maximum effect and there is no further change in the dose response relationship.

In the relationship E = α(DR), alpha (α) is a constant that can be determined experimentally to measure intrinsic activity. The significance of intrinsic activity is revealed by the study of *agonists* and *antagonists*. *Agonist* is that agent which produces an effect when it combines with the receptor. *Antagonists* are drugs which will reduce or abolish the effect of agonist. For the neurotransmitter acetylcholine (agonist) the antagonist can be atropine or tubocurarine which inhibits the effect of acetylcholine at the different cholinergic receptor sites. Some drugs like nalorphine can exhibit partial agonistic properties, because such drugs also possess some intrinsic activity.

Useful information about the character of recetpors have been derived from various studies of agonists versus antagonists. *An agonist* is an agent that produces a particular pharmacological action when it combines with a specific receptor. The function of the antagonist is the prevention of this effect.With the development of various synthetic antagonists different receptors could further be classified into specific subtypes accounting for a particular pharmacological action of an antagonist e.g. histamine receptors have been subtyped into H_1 and H_2 receptor and on the same lines muscarinic receptors into M_1, M_2 and M_3.

Antagonism by any drug at the receptor site can be either competitive or non-competitive. A compititive antagonist competes in a reversible manner for the same receptor site. To determine the nature of competition one has to determine the log dose-response of the agonist in presence of the antagonist. The competitive antagonist shifts the log dose response curve to the right and the E max of the agonist remains the same, only a higher concentration of agonist is required to achieve the same response as required in the absence of antagonist. Fig. 1.4 shows such a shift for any competitive antagonist where there is a parallel shift in the curve.

In non competitive antagonism the antagonist binds irreversibly to the receptor or to another site that inhibits the response to the agonist. In this case with an increase in the amount of agonist the action of antagonist is not neutralized.

This results in nonparallel shift of the log dose-response curve and lowering of E_{max} of the agonist in the presence of antagonist. Such an effect has been illustrated in Fig. 1.5

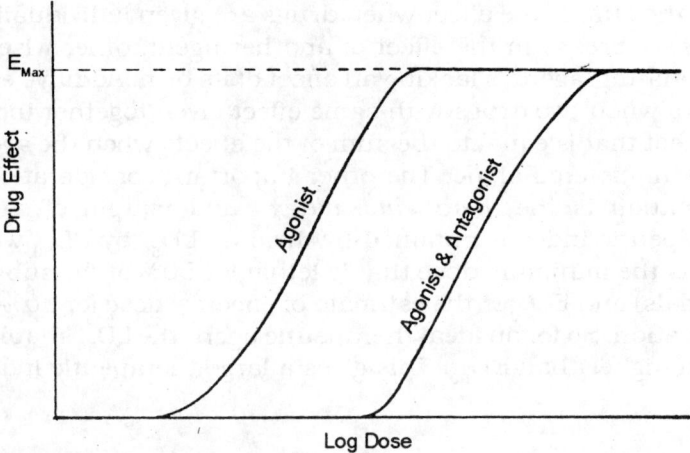

Fig. 1.4 : Log dose-response curve in presence of a completitive antagonist (parallel shift)

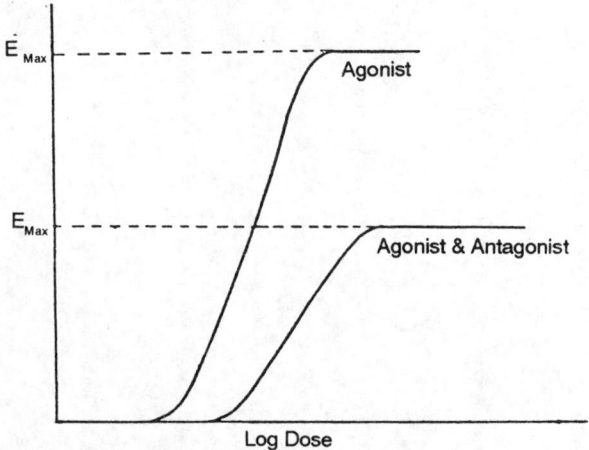

Fig. 1.5 : Non parallel shift of the log-dose response & lowering of E_{Max} by a non-competitive antagonist.

Administration of two different drugs at the same time sometimes show synergism, potentation or additive effects. All these terms relate to enhancement of drug effect. *Synergism* implies an effect that is greater in magnitude than the sum of the effect when drugs are given individually.

Potentiation implies an effect that is greater in magnitude than the sum of the effect when drugs are given individually. It implies increase in the effect of another agent, other wise the potentiating agent is lacking an effect of its own. Additive effect occurs when two drugs with same effect given together induce an effect that is equal to the sum of the effects when the agents are administered alone. The other important consideration in medication is the *therapeutic index* and margin of safety. Therapeutic index is obtained by dividing LD_{50} by ED_{50} where LD_{50} is the minimum dose that is lethal for 50% of the subjects (animals) and ED_{50} is the estimate of effective dose for 50% of a population. So for an ideal therapeutic agent the LD_{50} should be much higher than ED_{50}. This gives a large therapeutic index.

DRUGS ACTING ON THE
AUTONOMIC NERVOUS SYSTEM

The autonomic Nervous System is a portion of the nervous system concerned with the regulation of activity of cardiac muscle, blood vessels, smooth muscle and glands but is not subject to voluntary control and is functionally independent. In this system nerves and ganglia distribute efferent impulses to the heart, smooth muscles and glands and collect afferent impulses from them. It has two parts :

(a) Parasympathetic system

(b) Sympathetic system.

Parasympathetic System : The parasympathetic nerve fibers are contained in the cranial nerve and sacral pelvic nerves. The cranial nerves which are under parasympathetic control are oculomotor, facial, glossopharyngeal and the vagus.

Oculomotor nerve mediates contraction of the pupil and accommodation of the lens for near vision. The facial nerve carries the secretomotor and vasodilator impulse to the lacrimal, nasal and salivary glands. The glossopharyngeal nerve carries the fibers for taste from the tongue.

The Xth cranial nerve or vagus supplies the digestive tract, respiratory tract and the heart. The efferent fibers of the vagus are situated in terminal ganglia lying close or on the wall of the organ it supplies.

The parasympathetic nerve fbers control the involuntary function of the gastro intestinal system, urinary bladder, bronchi, salivary glands and the heart.

Sympathetic Nervous System

In this nervous system the preganglionic neurones are within the thoracic and lumbar portion of the spinal cord and the ganglionic fibers arise from cell bodies in the intermediolateral column of the spinal cord. They enter the sympathetic ganglia which lies close to this cord from where the post ganglionic fibers arise to innervate the blood vessels and viscera so that they are in control of the blood vessels, tone and other homoestatic functions.

2.1. DRUGS ACTING ON THE PARASYMPATHETIC SYSTEM (PARASYMPATHOMIMETIES)

In the parasympathetic division of the autonomic nervous system the neurotransmitter is acetylcholine, a chemical mediator that transmits impulses across the neural junction both at the pre and post ganglionic synaptic sites.

Drugs acting on parasympathetic system affect the interaction between the neuro transmitter and the receptor of the effector cell or cause enzymatic destruction of the neurotransmitter itself.

2.1.1 Acetylcholine (Ach)

It is a quarternary ammonium salt which undergoes rapid hydrolysis by plasma cholinesterase and therefore finds little therapeutic use.

However, acetylcholine can be used as a miotic in cataract surgery because it is a strong contractor of the iris muscle.

Pharmacological actions of acetylcholine : Acetylcholine produces a negative inotropic and chronotropic effect on the heart.

With small doses it produces vasodilation and fall in blood pressure which can be abolished by atropine. In animal experiments it can be demostrated that a large dose of Ach produces rise in blood pressure after adequate atropinization. This rise in blood pressure is attributed to the release of adrenaline from the adrenal medulla and activation of the sympathetic ganglia. This effect is known as the nicotinic action of Ach.

Acetylcholine increases the gastrointestinal motility and secretory activity. It produces contraction of smooth muscle in ureter, bladder and bronchioles. It stimulates the salivary, sweat and lacrimal glands. These are the muscarinic actions of Ach. These actions of acetylcholine can be best explained on the basis of the receptor theory according to which cholinergic receptors have been subdivided into two types,

(i) muscarinic and

(ii) nicotinic.

Receptors are transmembranous glycoproteins. On binding to a neurotransmitter or any agonist, the receptor is activated in a manner which its not understood at the molecular level. However pharmacologists have classified them according to the ligand which they bind. So it is implied that a receptor activated by an agonist of a given class will initiate a sequel of biological events which are unique for a type of ligand.

Thus the muscarinic acetylcholine receptors are further subtyped as M_1 and M_2. M_1 receptors have been sited in the autonomic ganglia and CNS. Typical M_1 agonist is Oxytremorine and the antagonist is pirenzepine. M_2 receptors are located at the end effector site. Typical M_2 agonist is Muscarine and the antagonist is Atropine.

Nicotinic acetylcholine receptors have been located in the autonomic ganglia and the skeletal muscles.

Nicotine, the alkaloid from tobacco is an agonist as well as an antagonist because it initially stimuates the receptor and then blocks it.

The *Nicotinic receptors* of the skeletal muscles are blocked by d-tubocurarine group of drugs which are used as muscle relaxants during anesthetic procedures. In the autonomic ganglia the nicotinic acetylcholine receptors are preferentially blocked by the Hexamethonium group of agents. They can be used as anti hypertensive drugs.

2.2. CHOLINERGICS RESISTANT TO CHOLINESTERASE (PARASYMPATHOMIMETICS)

This group of agents are not acted upon by cholinesterase or are hydrolysed at much slower rate so that they can have a longer duration of action with all the effects of acetylcholine.

The use of cholinergic agonist is contraindicated in coronary insufficiency, hypothyroidism, peptic ulcer and asthma. The representative parasympathomimetics are : Bethanechol Methacholine, Carbachol and Pilocarpine.

2.1.2.1. Bethanechol

It has predominant muscarinic effect and can be used in esophageal reflux, urinary bladder distension and other conditions. The usual dose is 10-20 mg. with meal.

2.1.2.2. Methacholine

Methacholine chloride in a dose of 10-25 mg through subcutaneous route produces all muscarinic actions of Ach with longer duration of action.

2.1.2.3. Carbachol

This agent is not readily succeptible to hydrolysis by cholinesterase. It has both muscarinic and nicotinic effects.

Carbachol is available as a an injectable in a dose of 0.25 to 0.5 mg.

It can be used as a 0.01% solution to produce miosis during ocular surgery.

2.1.2.4. Pilocarpine

This is an alkaloid. When applied locally to the eye it causes miosis and fall in intraocular pressure. It is mainly used in the treatment of glaucoma. Pilocarpine nitrate drops are used in the strength of 0.5% and 1 to 4% as the need may be. Miosis lasts for several hours.

Toxic effects of all these drugs are characterised by excessive parasympathomimetic actions on the cardiovascular system which is indicated by fall in blood pressure and slowing of the heart. There is increased salivation, nausea, vomiting and weakness.

2.3. PERIPHERALLY ACTING SYNTHETIC AGENTS ENHANCING ACH EFFECT AT THE MUSCARINIC SITE OF THE GASTROINTESTINAL TRACT (MODIFIERS OF GASTRO-DUODENAL MOTILITY).

Metoclopramide and Cisapride are the two representative drugs belonging to this group.

2.3.1. Metoclopramide Hydrocholride

This drug stimulates the upper gastrointestinal tract (GIT). It is a peripherally acting drug which enhances the action of Ach at the muscarinic sites of the GIT and stimulates motility. However, it does not stimulate gastric or pancreatic secretions. It also antagonizes dopamine in the CNS and probably this effect is responsible for its use as anti emetic agent.

It is used in delayed gastric emptying and gastro esophageal reflux.

The dose of the agent is 5 to 10 mg a day.

Metoclopramide is not to be concomitantly administered with phenothiazines, butyrophenones or thioxanthenes. It is contraindicated in pheochromocytoma and acute poryphyria (urinary excretion of porphobilinogen).

Untoward effects are impariment of power of voluntary movement and loss of muscle tone.

It causes prolactin secretion, galactorrhea and menstural disorders.

3.3.2. Cisapride

This agent is chemically related to metoclopramide but is devoid of dopamine blocking activity.

Cisapride enhances gastric motility. It is indicated in dyspepsia and impaired gastric emptying.

The dose is 5 mg three times a day. The drug is contraindicated in pregnancy and in children under twelve years of age.

It is metabolized by liver, so in abnormal liver function the dose is to be halved.

2.4. ANTICHOLINESTERASES

The group of drugs possessing anticholinesterase activity are *physostigmine. Neostigmine. Edrophonium. Pyridostigmine.*

organo-phosphate cholinesterase inhibitor like *Diisopropyll phosphoro-fluoride* (DFP) and insecticides like Parathion. These agents inhibit Ach hydrolysis so that more Ach is available at the neuroeffector junction where Ach is the transmitter.

2.4.1. Physostigmine (eserin)

It is an alkaloid obtained from calabar bean. It is well absorbed from the oral route, subcutaneous tissue and mucous membrane. However the drug gets cleaved by plasma esterases. Physostigmine forms reversible complex with cholinesterase at the site where Ach is broken down, so more Ach is available for its action. Physostigmine sulphate eye ointment and physostigmine salicylate eye drops are used for glaucoma to reduce intraocular pressure in the strength of 0.25%. The oral dose of physostigmine salicylate is 0.6 to 1.2 mg. It can be put to therapeutic use in atropine, phenothiazine and tricyclic antidepressent intoxication.

2.4.2. Neostigmine

This is a synthetic anticholinerterase. Neostigmine bromide (Prostigmin) can be used orally. However, it is poorly absorbed from the oral route. Effective parenteral dose is 0.5 to 2 mg. It is excreted in urine. Neostigmine is used for reversing the effect of non depolarising neuro muscular blocking agents. It is used in the management of paralytic ileus, atony of urinary bladder and myasthenia gravis. Myasthenia is a disorder of neuromuscular function thought to be due to the presence of antibodies of Ach receptor at the neuromuscular junction causing fatigue and exhaustion.

2.4.3. Pyridostigmine

It is a physostigmine like anticholinesterase mainly used in the treatment of myasthenia. The effective concentration for restoration of muscular strength in myasthemia gravis lies between 50-100 microgram of the drug in blood plasma, which can be obtained from an oral dose of 30 mg a day.

Pyridostigmine bromide tablets and sustained release tablets are available for oral administration.

2.4.4. Organophosphates

These cholinesterase inhibitors are represented by :

2.4.4.1. Disopropyl flurophosphate (DFP) is the typical compound which forms covalent bond between its phosphorus atom and the esteratic site of the cholinesterse. This enzyme-inhibitor complex is irreversible.

It therefore finds very little therapeutic use except in certain type of glaucoma.

2.4.4.2. Echothiopate is similar to DFP in its pharmacological action but spontaneous regeneration of phosphorylated enzyme can occur. Therefore its major use is in the treatment of glaucoma.

Echothiopate for ophthalmic use is marketed as powder, the solution is to be prepared fresh with a suitable diluent.

Untoward Effects : The untoward effect of DFP group of agents are miosis, increased bronchial secretion, profuse sweating, increased lacrimal secretion, anorexia, vomiting and diarrhea, bradycardia, anxiety, confusion and convulsion followed by vasomotor depression. Weakness of skeletal muscles especially those of respiration is seen. Symptoms of poisoning from insecticides like parathion are very much similar to those of untoward effects of DFP.

2.4.5. Pam (pyridine 2-aldoxine methyl chloride)

This drug reverses the effect of organophosphate anticholienesterase e.g. DFP as it combines with and splits off the phosphorous from the esteratic site so that the enzyme is again activated. With the reactivation of the enzyme accumulated acetylcholine begins to disappear. Treatment with PAM is required immediately because phosphorylated enzyme slowly changes to a form that cannot be reversed.

2.5. NEUROMUSCULAR BLOCKING AGENTS

These drugs are used in promoting muscle relaxation during general anesthesia. Two classes of drugs viz. depolarizing agents like Succinyl choline and non-depolarizing agents like Tubocurarine and Gallamine are used in clinical practice.

Mode of action of neuromuscular blocking agents : Acetylcholine is the neurotransmitter of the motor nerve. It reacts with the receptors at the muscle endplate to produce depolarization which means loss of charge. The depolarised end plate must get repolarised for normal propagation of nerve impulse across the neuromuscular junction. This is achieved by the enzymatic hydrolysis of liberated acetylcholine by the cholinesterase present at the motor endplate of the neuromuscular junction.

Depolarizing agents like succinylcholine which is administered as I.V. drip reacts with Ach receptors at the neuromuscular junction leading to persistent depolarisation of the excitable membrene although it produces muscle fasciculations. After prolonged exposure to the drug a reduction in receptor sensitivity occurs leading to flaccid paralysis of the skeletal muscle. The neuromuscular block by depolarizing agents like succinylcholine cannot be reversed by any other drug but it wears off in a very short time. So the duration of action is very short for such group of drugs. The mode of action of a competitive neuromuscular blocking agent like tubocurarine and galamine depends on their reversible combination with Ach receptors at the motor end plate of the neuromuscular junction. The number of available Ach receptors decreases so that the muscle threshold for excitation cannot be reached. Such blocks can be antagonised by increasing the concentration of Ach at the neuromuscular junction by the use of cholinesterase inhibitors like neostigmine.

Thus the advantage of competitive blockers like tubocurarine over succinylcholine is that the action of former can be reversed.

Side effects and untoward drug reaction

In persons deficient in serum cholinestarese succinylcholine's action is prolonged. Tubocurarine may produce dose related fall in blood pressure because of histamine release which can also cause bronchospasm. Galamine causes rise in blood pressure due to vagolytic and tyramine like effect. Gentamicine and other aminoglycoside antibiotics exert synergistic effect with neuromuscular blocking drugs. All inhalation anaesthetics increase the effect of neuromuscular blocking drugs.

2.6. PARASYMPATHETIC ANTAGONISTS

These drugs are used to relax smooth muscle. They can be obtained from natural sources or from synthetic sources.

Drugs from natural sources are Atropine and Scopolamine and are known as belladona alkaloids.

2.6.1. Atropine

This is an alkaloid obtained from Atropa belladona. Atropine produces its effect by the blockade of muscarinic receptors. It reduces the secretion in the upper and lower respiratory tract and so is useful as a preanesthetic agent. 0.5 mg to 1 mg produces inhibition of all secretions. Atropine antagonises the action of Ach in the central nervous system and thus shows antitremor activity via central antimuscarinic mechanism.

The drug is absorbed from the oral route but it can also be given parenterally. The oral dose lies between 0.25 to 1 mg given as atropine sulphate. Atropine decreases the frequency of peristaltic contractions and reduces the tone of stomach, small intestine and colon by virtue of its effect on involuntary muscle. It also relaxes the biliary tract, bladder and ureter tone.

On the basis of these effects it is used in the treatment of renal and biliary colic.

It is also useful in the treatment of poisoning by anticholinesterase and similar insecticides like parathion. Atropine blocks the Ach induced response to the ciliary muscles of the lens and circular smooth muscles of the iris. This effect produces cycloplegia and mydriasis which forms the basis for its opthalmic use. Toxic effect of atropine are rapid pulse, dilated pupil, dry mouth, raised body temperature and flushed skin, disorientation, restlessness and confusion. Physostigmine can be used as antidote.

Belladona alkaloids are rapidly absorbed from the oral route. Atropine has a half life of two and a half hours and most of it is excreted in urine within 12 hours as metabolites and partly unchanged.

2.6.2. Homatropine

This is a semi synthetic tropane alkaloid. It is a rapidly acting anti muscarinic agent exclusively used as cycloplegic and mydriatic agent in the form of eye drops (1-2% solution).

2.6.3. Hyoscine or Scopalamine

This is an alkaloid with similar therapeutic use and effects as those of atropine. Hyoscine is more effective in motion sickness. It is more potent than atropine in some of its antimuscaranic action with strong sedative effects. The effective dose of Hyoscine is 0.3 to 0.6 mg per day.

Synthetic anti-spasmodics : Methantheline, Propantheline and Dicyclomine are the representative agents.

2.6.4. Propantheline

It is used for the treatment of various kinds of smooth muscle spasm like bladder spasm and anuresis. The agent is effective in a dose of 15 mg every 6 hours. At higher dose it can produce neuromuscular blockade.

2.6.5. Dicyclomine

It is a synthetic antimuscarinic drug which decreases spasm in most smooth muscles without producing atropine like side effects on heart, eye or salivary glands. It is uded to decrease spasm of gastrointestinal tract, billiary tract in a dose of 20 mg every 4 hours. It is thought to have direct relaxant effect rather than competitive antagonism at the muscarinic receptors for Ach.

2.6.6. Methantheline, Oxyphenonium, Pipenzolate

Gastrointestinal effects of methantheline are greater than those of atropine and is more prolonged. The dose is 50-100 mg every 6 hourly.

The other compounds of this category are oxyphenonium bromide, which is indicated in infantile colic, gastrointestinal spasm at usual dose of 10mg and pipenzolate methyl bromide which has same indications as dicyclomine at 2.5-5mg dose 8 hourly.

Drugs acting on the sympathetic system (Adrenergic Agents): The sympathetic neurotransmitter is nor-adrenaline. This acts on the effector cell at the post ganglionic synapse whereas pre ganglionic synapse is activated by Ach with the exception of the sweat gland and some blood vessels where Ach acts as sympathetic transmitter.

Drugs that produce effect on the sympathetic system can :

(a) Affect the synthesis, storage, or release of the neurotransmitter.

(b) Affect the interaction between the neurotransmitter and the receptor or enzymatic destruction of the neurotransmitter.

Sympathomimetics or Adrenergic Agents : These drugs mimic the action of sympathetic stimulation. Two endogenous sympathomimetic agents Noradrenaline and Adrenaline produce various physological effects on the body systems to control involuntary homeostatic functions. Biosynthesis of noradrenaline and adrenaline occurs through the following pathways :

1. Tyrosine is hydroxylated by the enzyme hydroxylase to yield dihydroxy phenylalanine (DOPA).

2. DOPA is then decarboxylated to yield Dopamine.

3. Dopamine is hydroxylated at the beta carbon to yield nor-adrenaline.

4. Nor-adrenaline is methylated to form adrenaline and stored in the adrenal medulla. Also the dopamine formed in the above biosynthetic pathways enters the vesicle of the nerve terminal where it is converted to noradrenaline.

Release of the neurotransmitter occurs because of stimulation of the nerve terminal as a result of which depolarization takes place with the generation of action potential. In the next sequence the storage vesicle containing the neurotransmitter fuses with the plasma membrane as a result of which the neurotransmitter is released into the space between the nerve terminal and the effector organ.

Once set free from the nerve terminal the neurotransmitter noradrenaline activates the post synaptic receptors to produce various responses characteristic for each receptor type.

The action of noradrenaline is terminated by several mechanisms the most important of which is the reuptake of noradrenaline back into the nerve terminals. A portion of the noradrenaline so released is metablised by two enzymes viz. Catechol−O−methyl transferase (COMT) that acts upon noradrenaline which enters the cell and the noradrenaline in the exoplasm of the nerve terminal is metabolised by the enzyme monoamine oxidase (MAO) first into an aldehyde and then into glycol or to 3 methoxy 4 hydroxy mandelic acid (Vanillyl mandelic acid; VMA). VMA is the major metabolite excreted in the urine. The estimation of VMA in urine is important in diagnosis of pheochromocytoma and neuroblastoma.

Some important drugs affecting the sympathetic transmission act at specific steps of the biosynthesis and the disposition of noradrenaline to produce a particular therapeutic effect. For example :

(a) Conversion of DOPA to dopamine by dopa decarboxylase is inhibited by the agent alfa methyl dopa.

(b) Movement of dopamine into vesicles is inhibited by the alkaloid reserpine.

(c) Movement of noradrenaline back into vesicle is inhibited by reserpine.

(d) Release of noradrenaline by indirectly acting sympathominetics are blocked by cocaine and reserpine by depletion of the stores.

2.7. ADRENERGIC RECEPTORS

Sympathomimetic drugs initiate their effects by interaction with receptor macromolecules in or on the cells.

Receptors that are located in the plasma membrane of the cell may couple with specific effector molecules via intermediary coupling proteins. These coupling proteins are termed as "G" proteins as they bind and hydrolyze the guanine nucleotide.

Several distinct types of receptors for adrenergic drugs have been defined according to the chemical specificity of their ligand binding.

The adrenoceptor family have been classified into $Alfa_1$, $Alfa_2$, $Beta_1$, and $Beta_2$.

This pharmacological classification tells us little about the biological functions, $Alfa_1$ and $Alfa_2$ receptor subtypes and probably Beta-adrenoceptors can have multiple and diverse function which may be due to the fact that each receptor subtype couples to a different G protein.

However, it has been found that receptor subtypes are coupled to distinct effector pathways; Beta receptors stimulate the enzyme adenylate cyclase leading to generation of cyclic adenosine mono phosphate (CAMP). Similarly the $Alfa_1$ adrenergic receptors activate the enzyme phospholipase with guanine nucleotide regulatory proteins in the phospholipid visicles of the adrenergic receptors.

Location of adrenergic receptors : Alpha adrenergic receptors are located as follows :

(a) Alfa$_1$ adrenergic receptors are distributed post synaptically and are located on blood vessels, gastrointestinal tract, radial muscles of the eye and splenic capsule.

(b) Alfa$_2$ adrenergic receptors are distributed presynaptically and functionally they are inhibitory. When alfa$_2$ receptors are stimulated they inhibit further release of noradrenaline from the nerve terminal, so the adrenergic tone of the blood vessels are reduced :

Beta receptors are subdivided into two groups :

(a) Beta$_1$ that are located on the heart and intestine.

(b) Beta$_2$ are found on the bronchial and vascular smooth muscles.

2.7.1. Sympathomimetic Drugs

Adrenaline (Epinephrine) : The following are the pharmacological actions of adrenaline dependent on the type of receptors it reacts with in a particular tissue and site.

1. In low concentrations adrenaline will show beta$_2$ effects pre dominently, with relaxation of bronchiolor smooth muscle.

2. Large doses cause increase in systolic blood pressure more than diastolic pressure, mediated through activation of Alfa$_1$ receptors and increased ventricular contraction through the activation of Beta$_1$ receptors, causing increased cardiac output and increase in heart rate, with a compensatory vagal activity.

3. Adrenaline causes decreased cutaneous blood flow but increased blood flow to skeletal muscle.

4. Hepatic and renal blood flow decreases due to more vascular resistance.

5. Metabolic effects are increased through liver and muscle glycogenolysis. It is beta$_2$' receptor mediated. The other metabolic effect is an increase in free fatty acids, mediated through cyclic AMP.

Therapeutic Uses : It is not absorbed from the oral route. It is administered as subcutaneous injection in a dose of 0.5 mg in the treatment of bronchospasm in asthmatics.

It can restore cardiac activity in cardiac arrest. It is one of the primary drugs in the treatment of anaphylactic shock.

Adrenaline prolongs the action of local anaesthetics by cutaneous vaso-constriction.

It can be used to facilitate aqueous drainage in chronic open angle glaucoma.

2.7.2. Noradrenaline (Norepinephrine)

Noradrenaline is equipotent to adrenaline in its action on the $Beta_1$ receptor activation. However it has little effect on $Beta_2$ receptors. It is very potent $alfa_1$ agonist. Intravenous injection raises both systolic and diastolic pressure by constriction of vascular smooth muscle mediated through alfa receptors. So increased peripheral resistance results in compensatory vagal activity which slows the heart rate, cardiac output decreases but the coronary blood flow is increased.

Side Effects : Both the drugs can cause anxiety and head-ache. They can cause cardiac arrhythmias specially when concomitantly given with digitalis and some anaesthetic agents. It can cause pulmonary edema from pulmonary hypertension.

2.7.3. Dopamine

Dopamine is naturally occuring sympathetic amine which is the endogenous precursor of noradrenaline. Dopamine is often used for treating shock as it increases inotropy while also restoring perfusion to vital organs. It is used in low dosage for augmenting renal blood flow. Dopamine may preserve renal function in shock states. The half life of the agent is two to three minutes, It is administered as infusion to reach a steady state within 10 to 15 minutes. Infusion rate is linearly related to plasma concentration which is directly related to pharmacodynamic effect. At a low dose of less than 4 micro gm per kg per minute it activates dopamine receptors one and two, increasing renal blood flow, glomerular filtration rate and sodium excretion. Dopamine is a direct agonist of Beta one receptors at doses between 4 to 10 microgram per kg per minute resulting in increased heart rate and cardiac out put, by virtue of this action it is also indicated in chronic refractory congestive heart failure. A dose greater than 10 microgram per kg per minute results in excessive sympathetic stimulation so it can result into anginal pain and arrhythmias. However these effects are short lived because it is rapidly metabolised.

2.7.4. Dobutamine

Dobutamine resembles dopamine chemically but without its effect on dopaminergic receptors. It is a direct Beta-one receptor agonist and its inotropic effect is greater than chronotropic effect. It is used to improve myocardial function by raising cardiac output and stroke volume. Dobutamine improves myocardial oxygen supply and the oxygen demand of the heart remains less compared to other sympathomimetics because dobutamine causes minimal changes in heart rate and systolic blood pressure.

Dobutamine increases atrioventricular conduction so it can be used in atrial fibrillation.

Newer agents : Inotropic drugs which enhance systemic blood flow and provide renal protection but lack undesirable vasoconstrictor effects have led to the development of several novel dopaminergic agents.

Fenoldopam is a dopamine I receptor agonist with no alpha or beta effects. It is 10 times more potent at dopamine I receptors. It produces dose dependent reduction in systemic vascular resistance and blood pressure. Renal blood flow increases by 40 percent. *Ibopamin* is a compound which is metabolised to epinine, a dopamine I receptor agonist with some activity at alpha and beta receptors.

2.7.5. Phenylephrine

This sympathomymetic is used as a nasal decongesent and mydriatic. It is a directly acting sympathomymetic with its effect similar to noradrenaline but less potent with a longer duration of action.

Parenteral administration produces vasoconstriction, increased arterial pressure and reflex bradycardia. Adverse drug reaction are cardiac irregularities from a large dose. It is contraindicated with beta blockers as it increases the risk of cardiac irregularities and intracranial hemorrhage. Phenylephrine eye drops as 5% and 10% solution can be used as mydriatic. but is contraindicated in hyperthyroidism and narrow angle glaucoma.

2.7.6. Ephedrine

It is a mixed sympathomimetic amine having both direct and indirect action. It is absorbed when given orally but is not metabolised by COMT or MAO so the action is prolonged. The main use of drug is in the treatment of bronchial asthma in an oral dose which varies between 15 to 50 mg. Adverse drug reaction are CNS stimulation which produces insomnia, nervousness, nausea and agitation. It is contraindicated in hyperthyroidism and cardiovascular disease.

2.7.7. Amphetamine

It produces its effect by releasing noradrenaline. The dextrorotatory form is more potent in CNS stimulation. It depresses the appetite and decreases food intake by affecting the feeding center in the hypothalamus.

Tolerance to amphetamine occurs with in weeks of its use with psychic and physical dependence.

Adverse effects : Toxic psychosis, mental depression and fatigue. Amphetamine is contraindicated in cardiovascular diseases, in patients receiving MAO inhibitors or guanethidine because amphetamine increases noradrenaline concentration. Acute toxicity can be treated by acidification of urine with ammonium chloride administration. The CNS symptoms and the rise in blood pressure is treated with a dose of chlorpromazine because of its alfa receptor blocking effect. Other pharmacological effects of anphetamine is the stimulation of medullary respiratory center. It induces a decreased sense of fatigue, increased motor and speech activity with elevation of mood and increased alertness. For these reasons it is a drug of abuse.

2.7.8. Metaraminol

This agent is a sympathomimetic similar to noradrenaline in its action but less potent, with prolonged action. It has little CNS stimulant action. Metaraminol is absorbed from the oral route. However, parentral administration is more effective and is used in a dose of 2 to 10 mg after suitable dilution in the treatment of hypotension and shock. It induces sustained rise in both systolic and diastolic pressure with marked reflex slowing of the heart which can be prevented by atropine.

2.8. BETA ADRENERGIC AGENTS

Beta adrenergic drugs can be either an agonist or an antagonist to the beta adrenergic receptors.

Beta adrenergic receptors stimulate the enzyme adenylate cyclase leading to the generation of AMP coupled to guanine nucleotide regulatory proteins, Drugs find their therapeutic value if they are selective agonist or antagonist of this receptor subtype.

Beta-2-stimulating agents : Selective $Beta_2$ agonist have relaxing effect on the bronchial smooth muscles.

These agents are used as aerosol inhalants in the management of bronchial asthma. The metered valve delivers 100 micro gram per dose.

The following drugs are the representative bronchodilators: Salbutamol; Terbutaline; Metaproterenol; Albuterol; Bitolterol and Theophyllin.

2.8.1. Salbutamol

This is the most selective Beta-2 adrenergic stimulant. The effect appears within 2 to 3 minutes of inhalation and lasts for 4 to 6 hours.

Salbutamol is also used orally at a dose of 2 to 4 mg three times a day.

In emergencies salbutamol injection and respiratory solution can be used.

Side effect and contraindication : It may cause tremor of skeletal muscles. This effect is dose related. The drug is to be used with caution in patients of cardiac arrhythmias and other cardio-vascular complications. It also requires precaution in hyperthyroidism and in diabetes mellitus.

The other drugs which have similar pharmacological action as that of salbutamol with the following differences are :

2.8.2. Terbutaline

It has a longer duration of action, the dose being 250 micro gm. per metered dose.

2.8.3. Betolterol

It is a prodrug which is converted in the lung to colterol the active agent, with a longer duration of action than salbutamol or terbutaline.

2.8.4. Isoprenaline

This drug is not a specific Beta2 stimulating agent. It has also beta1 stimulating effect. It increases the heart rate and produces other sympathomimetic effects. The dose is 20 mg which can be given sublingully to give immediate effect. It is not to be given to children. The.drug is contra indicated in hypertension, coronary artery disease, diabetes, renal and hepatic failure.

2.9. XANTHINE DERIVATIVES

Theophylline and aminophylline are the Xanthine derivatives that are used in the treatment of asthma both for long term prophylaxis and acute attack.

They inhibit degradation of 3-5 cyclic AMP by interfering with phosphodiesterase activity.

It is not possible to establish a single dose regimen for theophylline and its derivatives that will suit all patients because the metabolism of theophylline varies greatly from person to person.

This variation is reflected in its elimination half life, which may vary from 4 hours to about 25 hours in patients.

Factors responsible for the variation are age, body weight, diet, concomitant illness and drug interactions.

2.9.1. Aminophillin

Aminophillin is theophylline ethylene diamine containing about 85% anhydrous theophylline. It is administered as tablets, injections, sustained release preparations.

2.9.2. Choline Theophyllinate

The other preparations are *choline theophyllinate* containing 64% anhydrous theophylline.

The factors responsible for the variation in the elimination half life of the theophyline group of drugs are age, body weight, diet, concomitaqnt illness and drug interactions. The therapeutic: toxic ratio for theophylline is very small. So only by measuring the plasma theophylline concentration the dosage are to be tailored.

Theophylline can be detected rapidly by an enzyme linked or fluoresent immunoassay.

Bronchodilation by theophylline depends upon critical blood level. Serum concentration of 10 to 20 micro gram per ml is required to produce adequate bronchodilation without producing the side effects. The usual dose is 150 to 200 mg given orally every 6 hours.

The side effects of theophylline are nausea, insomnia, dirrhoea, persistent vomiting, cardiovascular complications which are encountered with the rise in theophylline concentration in the blood.

The following drugs are likely to affect the plasma theophylline concentration. the drugs that increase the plasma concentration are :

Allopurinol, cimetidine, erythromycin and oral contraceptives whereas the drugs that reduce the concentration in plasma are δ Phenobarbitone, phenytoin, rifampin and sulphinpyrazone.

The adrenergic antagonists, the alfa adrenergic blockers and the beta adrenergic blocking agents have been considered along with antihypertensive agents in Chapter 3.

3

DRUGS ACTING ON THE CARDIOVASCULAR SYSTEM

Cardiovascular drugs can be grouped into the following subclasses depending on their specific therapeutic application.

(a) Cardiac Glycosides

(b) Antiarrhythmic and Antianginal drugs

(c) Drugs used in hypertension.

3.1. CARDIAC GLYCOSIDES

Digoxin and Digitoxin are cardiac glycosides obtained from leaves of the plant Digitalis lanata. Their specific use is in congestive heart failure and in slowing the ventricular rate in the supraventricular arrhythmias. Both the glycosides have similar pharmacological effects but different pharmacokinetic properties. The digitalis glycosides enhance the force of systolic contraction and increase the mechanical efficiency of failing heart and thus are used in treating congestive heart failure (CHF). These glycosides increase the force of myocardial contraction, slow down conduction, increase the vagal tone and prolong the refractory period of the auriculo ventricular node. Digitalis increases the cardiac output in patients with CHF. There is a reduction in reflex vasoconstriction because of improved circulation. So with improved myocardial contraction and decreased sympathetic activity more blood flows through the kidney to give diuretic effect of the glycosides.

Pharmacokinetic differences between Digoxin and Digitoxin

3.1.1. Digoxin

Only 70 percent of the oral dose is absorbed of which 30 percent is protein bound. The $t_{1/2}$ is about 36 hours. It is excreted slowly and therefore can accumulate in the body to reach a toxic level. The serum therapeutic concentration lies between 0.5 to 2.5 ng/ml of the blood. Any value exceeding 3 ng/ml will be toxic so drug monitoring by rapid assaying of plasma digoxin will help to reduce the dose and chances of toxicity.

3.1.2. Digitoxin

90 percent of digitoxin is absorbed from the gastro intestinal tract of which 97 percent of the drug is protein bound. The $t_{1/2}$ is very long which can be about 5 days. It is metabolized by the liver and the serum therapeutic concentration lies between 10 to 35 ng/ml of blood. Its metabolism is increased by hepatic microsomal inducers like phenobarbitone and phenytoin.

Administration of digitalis preparations is done by giving a loading dose and then a divided dose till digitalization. After optimal benifit 10 percent of the digitalization dose is given as a maintenence dose. Digitalis has a low margin of safety so blood level higher than the desired amount gives rise to toxic manifestations which can be fatal.

Digitalis glycoside intoxication may precipitate due to various reasons such as

  (i) Concomitant administration of potassium depleting diuretics

  (ii) Administration of the glycoside over a long period;

 (iii) Protracted vomiting and diarrhohea which causes potassium loss.

 (iv) Prolonged administration of corticosteroids

  (v) Hypothyroidism,

 (vi) Decreased renal function results in accumulation of the glycoside. Signs of digitalis toxicity are anorexia, vomiting, headache, fatigue, malaise, neuralgias, delirium and abnormal colour perception.

The toxic effects of digitalis can lead to ventricular and atrial arrhythmias. The untoward effects can be treated by discontinuing the drugs. Depending upon the serum potassium level it may be supplemented. Phenytoin can be given to treat ventricular and atrial arrhythmias. Atropine can be given to treat sinus bradycardia induced by digitalis toxicity.

3.2. OTHER DRUGS IN THE TREATMENT OF CHF

CHF can be treated with diuretics alone with sodium restriction which should not exceed 2 grams per day in the diet.

Vasodilators can be used in patients when digitalis and diuretics fail. Vasodilators decrease the preload and afterload. Dilators of the arteriole decrease the afterload and the venodilators reduce preload. The decrease in pre and afterload increases the cardiac out put and also decreases the pulmonary congestion. Vasodilator drugs that can be used are Hydralazine upto 200 mg t,d,s, Prazosin, and Captopril.

The pharmacological properties of these drugs have been given in the section of drugs used in the treatment of hypertension.

Antiarrhythmic Agents : These drugs are used in the treatment of cardiac arrhythmias. Features of cardiac arrhythmia are abnormalities in the rate and origin of cardiac impulse. So conduction disturbance of the normal sequence of activation of the atria and ventricles occurs.

The heart has a group of cells that can be self excited. The impulse so generated propagates to the rest of the heart. This group of cells are known as *pacemakers*. The normal pacemekers are situated at the sino-atrial node (SA node) and the latent pacemakers are situated at the atrio-ventricular node (AV node) and in the Purkinje fibres. The function of the pacemaker cells is to excite the heart and the electrical impulse required to excite it is termed as excitability. In normal conditions there is a minimal time interval between two electrical impulses generated from the pacemaker cells which is referred as *effective refractory period* (ERP).

When cardiac cells are excited a complex sequence of voltage change occurs as a function of time. The resting transmembrane voltage relative to the extracellular fluid is about - 90mv because of the concentration gradient for Na+ and K+ ions. Whenever the cardiac cell is excited there is a change in ionic conductance across the membrane with the generation of action potential and for a cardiac cell the ERP is related to action potential duration.

The heart cells have the ability to generate impulse spontaneously. This self regulating property is known as automaticity. Abnormality of this property alters the rhythm of the heart. Antiarrhythmic drugs depress the automaticity which results in decrease of the excitability of the pacemaker cells and thus increase the ratio between ERP over the action potential duration.

3.3. ANTIARRHYTHMIC DRUGS

Quinidine : This is the dextro stereoisomer of the alkaloid quinine, used in the treatment of supraventricular and ventricular arrythmias. It reduces the transmembrane voltage in atrial, ventricular and Purkinge fibres to affect the action potential sequence and increase ERP in these tissues. Quinidine has anticholinergic effect which can also contribute to its action on the heart. It also produces alfa receptor blockade with reduction in peripheral resistance resulting in a fall in blood pressure which is more prominent when given intravenously. The oral dose of the drug is 200 to 300mg three or four times a day. Maximum effect is seen with in one to two hours of oral administration, however 80 percent of the drug is bound to the plasma albumin.

Drug interactions : Quinidine increases the serum level of digitalis and thus can induce digitalis toxicity. Phenobarbital and phenytoin can shorten the duration of action of Quinidine because they increase the elimination rate. Quinidine can potentiate the vasodilator effects of nitroglycerin.

Adverse reactions : Nausea, vomiting, diarrhea and abdominal pain are the gastrointestinal effects. It can produce cinchonism which includes tinnitus (ringing in ear), loss of hearing and blurring of vision.

Procainamide : The effect of procainamide on the heart is similar to that of quinidine as it also decreases the action potential duration and ERP in atria and ventricles. It is used in the treatment of different types of arrhythmias.

Procainamide requires an effective plasma concentration of 3 to 10 µg/ml of blood to produce antiarrhythmic action which can be obtained from an oral dose of 200 to 500 mg. It is rapidly metabolized and takes about ½ hour to produce the peak effect. 15% of the drug is protein bound and is eliminated through liver and kidney. It is acetylated before excretion although 50 to 60 percent of the drug is excreted unchanged.

Adverse effects are cardiac depression and can precipitate glaucoma and urinary retention

Drug interactions: It enhances the effect of some beta-blockers. Cimetidine and amidoarone can enhance the effect of procainamide.

Disopyramide : Like quinidine it has both direct and indirect effect on the heart but only used in ventricular arrhythmias. Disopyramide in comparison to quinidine produces greater reduction of conduction velocity of the depolarization phase in the action potential sequence. The extra cardiac effect can be attributed to its atropine like action. About 83 percent of the drug is absorbed from the oral route of which 50 percent is excreted unchanged in the urine. The half life of the drug is 5 to 7 hours. The usual oral dose lies between 400 to 800mg a day.

Drug interaction : It can enhance the effect of some beta-blockers, if administered concomitantly.

Adverse effects : Hypotension and anti cholinergic effects like dry mouth, blurred vision.

Lidocaine : This is a local anesthetic administered intravenously as infusion in a dose of 1 to 1.5 mg/kg body weight to treat ventricular arrhythmia. The drug affects the duration of action potential and refractoriness due to the blockade of sodium current in the action potential sequence. Lidocaine under-goes extensive hepatic metabolism so it is not given orally. 70 percent of the drug is bound to the plsma proteins.

Adverse effects : drowsiness, convulsion and respiratory arrest.

Phenytoin : Phenytoin is an anti epileptic agent which is also effective in cardiac arrhythmias. Its cardiac electrophysiological actions are similar to that of lidocaine. Phenytoin is used in ventricular arrhythmias. It may be useful in arrhythmias associated with digitalis toxicity or in myocardial infraction. Phenytoin is administered orally with an initial loading dose of 15 mg/kg body weight followed by a maintenance dose of 4 mg/ kg body weight. The absorption of phenytoin is slow by the oral route. It is inactivated by the liver enzymes and is 90% protein bound. However plasma $t_{1/2}$ is prolonged with increasing dose. Phenytoin can be given as intravenous injection for the control of arrhythmias in a dose of 100mg intermittently.

Adverse effects : Drowsiness, nystagmus (spasmodic oscillatory movement of the eye), vertigo, ataxia and other neurological effects are usually seen when the plasma concentrations are high.

Propranolol : This is a beta adrenergic blocking drug used in hypertension and angina. It blocks the beta receptors in the sinus node inhibiting the sympathetic influence. This property makes it useful as an antiarrhythmic agent. It increases the effective refractory period and changes the duration of action potential. Blood concentration of propranolol is associated with its therapeutic effect. It should be between 20 to 1000 µg/ml depending upon the type of arrhythmia being treated. The drug is metabolized by the liver Its elimination decreases if the hepatic blood flow becomes less.

Adverse effects : It induces bronchospasm in asthmatics. Sudden withdrrawal can produce angina and severe hypertension.

Bretylium : Bretylium is used in a dose of 5 to 10 mg/kg as interavenous infusion to treat arrhythmias that are not controlled by other drugs. This is a adrenergic neuron blocking agent with a direct electrophysiologic effect on the heart. The oral absorption is poor so it is administered parenterally. It is excreted unchanged in urine and elimination half life is between 6 to 10 hours.

Adverse effect : Orthostatic hypotension.

Amiodarone : This is an iodinated benzofuran derivative used in ventricular arrhythmias which are refractory to other drugs. Amiodarone is used to increase the effective refractory period in the ventricle and auricles, to induce anti arrhythmic action. It has alfa and beta adrenergic blocking properties and therefore causes both systemic and coronary vasodilation

It is highly lipid soluble and its half life is more than ten days. It is used in a dose of 200 mg three times a day.

Drug interactions : It increases the serum level of digitalis, diltiazim, quinidine and procainamide. So concomitant treatment with these drugs require dose adjustments.

Adverse side effects :   Causes hyper- or hypo- thyroidism contraindicated in thyroid dysfunction. The other adverse effects are photosensitivity, ataxia, tremor and neuropathy.

3.4. ANTI ANGINAL DRUGS

Angina pectoris is the pain that results from ischemic heart disease. The primary drugs used are the coronary vasodilators. Various other group of drugs can also be used to treat such conditions e.g. beta-adenergic blockers, calcium channel modulators.

Nitrates : These are potent coronary vasodilators.

Nitrates cover the group of agents which are either esters of nitrous acid or poly esters of nitric acid. Nitroglycerine (Glyceryl trinatrate) is the prototype of this group.

Amylnitrite : It is a volatile liquid administered as inhalation in a dose.of 0.3 ml. Amyl Nitrite is a liquid consisting chiefly of the nitrites of 3-methylbutanol and 2-methylbutanol esterified with nitrous acid fraction of fusel oil. It is stored in a cool place protected from light.

Glyceryl Trinitrate : It is a volatile substance administered in small tablet form. The tablet is prepared with a suitable base and a solution of known amount of glyceryl trinitrate in ninety percent alcohol. It is kept in a tightly sealed container so that it does not lose its activity. Active drug produces distinct sensation when placed under the tongue. The dose of the drug is 0.5 to Img.

Glyceryl trinitrate can also be used as an ointment for topical administration in a strength of 2 per cent for controlling nocturnal angina which occurs during sleep. Transdermal nitroglycerine disc can be applied once in 24 hours to produce continuous concentration of the drug in blood for prophylaxis in angina pectoris. The other nitrates are *Isorbid dinitrate, pentaerythritol tetranitrate and Erythrityl tetranitrate.* These can be used as sustained release tablets in the strength of 40mg for 6 to 12 hourly dose and 80 mg for 12 hourly use. Erythrityl tetranitrate can be used as sublingual tablets in a dose of 5 to 10 mg three times a day.

3.4.1. Mode of Action of Nitrates

Organic nitrates are boitransformed into nitrite ions by reductive hydrolysis in the liver by the enzyme glutathion reductase. This enzyme converts the lipid soluble drug into the active water soluble metabolite which produce the effect. This biotransformation determines the duration of action for the organic nitrates. Nitroglycerine reacts with glutathione to release inorganic nitrite ions. Nitroglycerine peak plasma concentration is reached in four minutes after sublingual administration and with a half life of 1 to 3 minutes where as the metabolite, although less potent, appears to have 40 minutes half life.

The kinetics of hepatic reductive hydrolysis is different for each nitrate, which is influenced by the blood flow through the liver. In anginal attack the objective is rapid onset of action rather than longer duration of action so sublingual route is the route of choice as this gives effective concentration of the drug in circulation within minutes. However for long term treatment sustained release formulation can be used for slow onset and longer duration of action. Nitrates relax all smooth muscles including the vascular smooth muscles. They reduce the venous tone thereby increasing venous capacitance and decrease the venous return to the heart. At the same time reduction in peripheral arteriolar resistance by these agents can reduce the myocardial oxygen requirements. The venous dilation produces increased peripheral pooling of the blood. This causes decrease in the end diastolic volume and pressure. Simultaneously there is a decreased myocardial wall tension as a result of which there is less of oxygen requirement of the heart.

Nitrates produce vasodilation of the cerebral blood vessles with the increase in cerebral pressure which can cause headache. They also relax bronchial and biliary smooth muscles.

Adverse effects : These drugs when present in large amount can produce methemoglobinemia, headache and dizziness.

The other drugs that are used prophylactically to decrease the severity and frequency of anginal attacks are beta-adrenergic blocking drugs and calcium channel blockers.

3.5. BETA-ADRENERGIC BLOCKING DRUGS

The beta blockers oxprenolol, sotalol and propranolol are the commonly used drugs, however, these are not to be used in variant angina which is caused by coronary vasospasm. They are contraindicated in bronchospasm and asthma.

Pharmacological features of this group of drugs have been considered with anti hypertensive drugs.

3.6. CALCIUM CHANNEL BLOCKERS

This group of drugs have different therapeutic indications. The prototype agents are Verapamil, Nifedipine, Diltiazim, Amlopidine and Felodipine.

Verapamil : It was originally considered to be a potent coronary vasodilator for use in angina pectories. Now it is mainly indicated in cardiac arrhythmias. Verapamil decreases action potential amplitude, Prolongs the effective refractory period and affects conduction in AV node via slow calcium ion channel modulation. It is used in the treatment of paroxysmal supraventricular tachycardia in an oral dose of 40 to 80 mg four times a day. It is contraindicated in cardiogenic shock, bradycardia, hepatic impairment and pregnancy.

Nifedipine : Nifedipine produces its anti anginal effect by modulation of calcium ion influx by selective inhibition. This prevents coronary artery spasm. Nifedipine reduces coronary vascular resistance and increases coronary blood flow. It can dilate coronary arteries in a small dose which does not reduce myocardial contractility. NIfedipine also exerts a potent vasodilator action on peripheral arterial bed. So it can be used in control of hypertension. The dose is 10 mg every 6-8 hrs. Nifedipine is almost fully absorbed after oral administration. Action appears within 20 to 45 minutes and lasts for 6 hours. 80 percent of the drug is excreted as metabolites in urine.

The side effects are headache, dizziness, flushing, hypotension and ankle oedema.

Diltiazim : The mode of action of diltiazim is similar to nifedipine. it is used in a dose of 30mg four times a day for angina. It is also indicated in vasospastic angina, in mild to moderate hypertension and as a prophylaxis of paroxysmal supraventricular tachyarrhythmias. However the doses for these conditions are 180 to 240 mg a day in divided doses.

Adverse drug interactions : Diltiazim is associated with depression of cardiac conduction particularly seen with concurrent treatment with beta blockers and digitalis. H_2 blockers may increase the plasma concentration of the drug and diltiazim also increases the cyclosporine plasma levels.

Amlodipine besylate : This is a calcium antagonist with less incidence of reflex tachycardia. It is used in hypertension, chronic stable angina and varient angina. The recommended dose is 5 to 10 mg daily. Its half life is prolonged in impaired liver function. It is highly protein bound.

Adverse effects : Muscle cramp, fatigue, dyspepsia and an over dose could result in severe hypotension.

Felodipine : It is a vasoselective calcium antagonist indicated in hypertension. It has natriuretic effect with no effect on cardiac conduction. It is contraindicated in pregnancy and nursing mother.

Drug interactions : Felodipine requires dose adjustment when it is prescribed with enzyme inducers e.g. phenytoin, carbamazepine and barbiturates as they decrease the plasma levels of felodipine. Dosage of the drug should be adjusted in individual patients. The recommended dose is 5 mg a day.

Side effects : Dose dependent ankle swelling, flushing, palpitation, dizziness and fatigue are common.

3.6.1. Nimodipine

This is a new class of calcium channel blocker which inhibits the contraction of smooth muscle. It acts primarily on the cerebral blood vessels exerting an anti-vasoconstrictive and anti-ischaemic action. The drug is used for prevention of ischaemic neurological disorders due to cerebral circulatory deficits. The recommended oral dose is 60 mg, 4 hourly.

Nimodipine is administered in a dose of I mg an hour as a slow intravenous infusion to treat ischaemic neurological defects in acute cerebral circulatory disorders since it dilates the cerebral blood vessels and improves the circulation. The drug is metabolised by the liver, and excreted in the urine.

Contraindications : Nimodipine is not to be used in cerebral oedema and in raised intracranial pressure. The drug should not be used with other calcium channel blockers like nifedipine. diltiazim and verapamil.

Concomitant administration of beta blockers should be avoided.

Side effects : The reported side effects are decrease in blood pressure, increase in heart rate, flushing, gastrointestinal disorders and nausea.

3.7. DIURETICS AND ANTI HYPERTENSIVE AGENTS

Essential hypertension and its etiology is still unknown therefore drug therapy is generally emperic and nonspecific. Maintenance of normal blood pressure is a function of a number of physiological and metabolic responses that control the stimulation of the autonomic nerves. This in turn controls the heart rate, the blood circulation through the kidney to maintain the blood volume and its composition and the peripheral resistance of the blood vessels.

The classes of drugs most commonly used for the control of hypertension are :

1. Diuretic agents
2. Beta blockers
3. Centrally acting sympatholytic agents
4. Post ganglionic adrenergic neuron blockers
5. Renin-angiotensin antagonist
6. Arterial and venous vasodilators and calcium channel blockers
7. Alfa adrenergic blocking drugs.

All these drugs have different sites and mechanism of action therefore they can be used in combination to combat several aspects of the pathophysiology of the disease. Hypertension is indicated whenever the systolic-diastolic blood pressure exceeds 140 and 90 mm of Hg respectively. Drug therapy is intended to bring down this elevated pressure to the normal range. This can be brought about by various agents, e.g. diuretics reduce the circulating blood volume, however their anti hypertensive effect, is due to saluresis and vasodilation. Increased adrenergic activity in hypertension can be reduced by use of specific adrenergic blockers like the centrally acting sympatholytic agents, beta adrenergic blockers, alfa adrenergic antagonists, adrenergic neuron blockers and sympathetic ganglion blocking drugs. All these groups of drugs reduce adrenergic drive on the heart and blood vessels. Vasodilators like calcium channel blockers and hydralazine group of drugs reduce the peripheral resistance offered by the blood vessels which results in their anti-hypertensive effect.

3.7.1. Diuretic Drugs

Hypertension and excessive fluid retention is treated with a diuretic. These agents promote loss of water and body salts with an increase in urine flow. Individual diuretics act on different parts of the nephron to exert their effect. They can be classified on the basis of their site of action as follows.

(i) **Osmotic diuretics** act on the proximal part of the tubule. The prototype is Mannitol.

(ii) **Thiazide** and related agents act on the first half of the distal convoluted tubule and on a portion of the cortical ascending limb of the loop of Henle. The prototype agents are Hydrochlorthiazide and Chlorthiazide.

(iii) **Loop diuretics** act in the ascending limb of Henle's loop. The representative agent is Furosemide.

(iv) **Aldosterone antagonist** act on the distal half of the convoluted tubule and the cortical portion of the collecting duct of the nephron. The prototype drug is Spironolactone.

(v) **Potassium sparing diuretic** agents act at the distal tubule of the nephron. The prototype agent is Triamterene.

The selection of a diuretic depends on the disease state of the individual.

(i) Osmotic diuretic

Mannitol, a six carbon sugar is administered intravenously in 10 or 20 percent solution as it is not absorbed orally. Mannitol is used in acute renal failure, management of hemolytic transfusion reactions, severe traumatic injury and incardiovascular operations. They are also used to reduce cerebrospinal fluid pressure.

Mannitol produces its effect at the proximal part of the tubule by decreased reabsorption of sodium and water thereby resulting in a large volume of urine.

(ii) Thiazide and related drugs

Hydrochlorthiazide and Chlorthiazide are the representative diuretics that are well absorbed by the oral route. Their peak action is seen in four hours and diuresis persists for about twelve hours. Thiazide diuretics reduce the reabsorption of sodium and chloride ions in the first half of the distal convoluted tubule and in a portion of the cortical ascending limb of the loop of Henle. So it produces urine with unabsorbed salt or increased excretion of sodium. Sodium -potassium ion exchange is enhanced and kaliuresis results. Thiazides are effective in the treatment of heart failure as long as glomerular filtration rate is more than 50 percent of the normal. The effective dose for hydrochlorthiazide is 50 to 100 mg a day.

Side effects for thiazides Potassium depletion and metabolic alkalosis. Metabolic alkalosis occur due to hydrogen ion secretion as a substitute for depleted stores of potassium. There is increased proximal tubular reabsorption of filtered bicarbonate ions (HCO_3^-) with a relative depletion of the extracellular fluid. Loss of potassium can be prevented by supplementing potassium. The other side effects of thiazides is the reduction in uric acid excretion which may lead to hyperuricemia. Granulocytopenia and hyperphosphatemia have also been reported as side effects of thiazides.

Chlorthiazide is administered in a dose upto 500 mg every six hourly. Other drugs that are available belonging to this group are *Chlorthalidone* and *Indapamide*. They differ principally in dosage and duration of action with very few significant advantages over the parent drug.

(iii) Loop diuretics

Furosemide, Bumetanide, Ethacrynic acid are the examples of loop diuretics with similar pharmacological action but with different chemical structures. These agents inhibit the reabsorption of sodium, potassium and chloride in the ascending limb of the Henles loop, possibly by blocking a transport system in the luminal membrane, they may also induce vasodilation in the renal cortex and can produce high rates of urine formation. Other diuretic agents lose their effectiveness as the blood volume tends to be normal whereas loop diuretics remain effective even after the elimination of excessive extracellular fluid volume. The urine formation may be as high as 1/4th of the glomerular filtration rate. All these properties make them high ceiling diuretics. Furosemide, Bumetanide and Ethacrynic acid are effective orally but can be given intravenously for quick effect. They are excreted in bile and urine. Oral dose for fursemide is between 40 to 80 mg a day.

This group of drugs can be used in heart failure particularly in pulmonary edema and refractory heart failure when response to ordinary treatment is inadequate. Furosemide can potentiate the action of thiazide, mannitol and spironolactone.

Adverse effects of loop diuretics is because of their diuretic potency. They can produce circulatory collapse and azotemia because of excess urea or other nitrogenous compounds in blood. Like the thiazides they can induce metabolic alkalosis because of large increase in excretion of chloride, hydrogen and potassium ions and induce hypokalemia and hyponatremia. The reabsorption of free water is also decreased.

(iv) Aldosterone antagonists

Spironolactone is the prototype drug of this group which structurally resembles aldosterone. Spironolactone produces its effect by acting on the distal tubules and collecting duct of the nephron; more sodium is excreted with the retention of potassium. This is more effective when the circulating aldesterone level is high, however the efficacy is not lost even when the serum concentration of aldosterone is within normal range. The drug is administered in a dose range of 25 to 100 mg three or four times a day. It is used in combination with thiazide or loop diuretics to reduce the loss of potassium. It is contraindicated in patients with hyperkalemia or hyponatremia and in renal failure.

It can be used in adrenal gland tumor to counteract the increased aldosterone level.

Adverse effects are nausea, epigastric distress, mental confusion drowsiness and gynecomastia and fluid or electrolyte imbalance.

Drug interactions : It increases the blood level of digoxin and

and reduces the effect of warfarin. It inhibits ulcer healing properties of carbenxolone.

(v) Potassium sparing diuretics

Triamterene and Amiloride are the prototype drugs. They produce their effect by blocking sodium reabsorption and inhibiting potassium secretion in the distal tubules of the nephron. Both drugs cause a moderate increase in excertion of sodium chloride and bicarbonate ions. These actions are similar to those of spironolactone but the action is independent of aldosterone because they have been found to be effective in adrenalectomized animals. The effective dose is 100mg once or twice a day for triamterene and 5 mg a day for amiloride. The two agents are effective in preventing potassium loss when administered with thiazides, so such combinations are useful in patients who develop hypokalemia with thiazide group of diuretics.

Drug interactions : Nonsteroidal anti inflammatory drugs may diminish the anti-hypertensive effect of these drugs. They can induce hyperkalaemia with other potassium sparing drugs and with potassium supplement.

Adverse effects are fluid and electrolyte inbalance, vomiting, abdominal pain, skin rash, postural hypotension, visual changes and muscle cramp.

3.8. BETA BLOCKERS

Beta adrenergic blocking drugs can be classified into the following subgroups.

(a) Non selective antagonist prototype drugs are propranolol and Timolol.

(b) Selective beta-I adrenergic antagonist drugs are Metoprolol, Atenolol and Betaxolol.

(c) Non selective but also with alfa adrenergic blocking action prototype is Labetalol.

(d) Non selective antagonist with intrinsic alfa adrenergic activity, Acebutol and Pindolol.

Therapeutic Uses : Beta adrenergic blockers find their use in hypertension incombination with other agents such as diuretics or other anti hypertensive agents. They can be used for prophylaxis in angina and management of arrhythmia. They are also indicated in hyoperthyroidism to reduce tachycardia. Beta blockers have also been used in migraine. Beta blocking agents are useful in the treatment of chronic open angle glaucoma and ocular hypertension, following topical application to the eye. Pharmacological profile of some individual beta adrenergic blocking drugs are as below;

Propranolol

This drug blocks both beta one and beta two adrenergic receptors. Propranolol decreases the heart rate and cardiac out put and prolongs systole. The coronary blood flow and the oxygen consumption by the cardiac tissue are decreased. Propranolol also inhibits secretion of renin which may also play a part in its anti hypertensive effect. Propranolol increases airway resistance so it cannot be used in asthmatics. Selective beta adrenergic antagonists like atenolol are indicated in such cases. Propranolol also augments hypoglycemic action of insulin. Propranolol is effective in 40 to 80 mg in divided doses. It is completely absorbed from the oral route and 90 percent of the drug is bound to the plasma proteins. It is metabolised by the liver into different metabolites of which 4 hydroxy propranolol is an effective antihypertensive with a shorter half life.

Drug interactions of all beta blockers are more or less common. They may enhance effects of calcium channel blockers such as verapamil. They enhance cardiac depressant effects of anaesthetics like halothane and the local anesthetic lignocaine, and antiarrythemics like quinidine and procainamide.So concomitant administration of these drugs requires caution.

Indomethacin may decrease effectiveness of propranolol. *Adverse effects* of beta blockers are cold extremites, sleep disturbances, fatigue, dizziness, bradycardia, confusion, bronchospasm, skin rash, dry eyes, impaired sexual function.

Timolol

It is a non selective beta blocking agent which is 5 to 10 times more potent than propranolol. It has a special pharmacological effect by virtue of which it can lower intraocular pressure by reducing production of aqueous humor with out change of pupil size or affecting the vision. Timolol drops in a concentration of

0.25 to 0.5 percent are used in chronic angle glaucoma in a dose of one drop twice a day or as required. The side effects are similar to those of other beta blockers.

Atenolol and Metoprolol

These two agents are selective beta adrenergic antagonists. They are the drugs of choice in the treatment of hypertension of asthmatics or elderly hypertensives with reduced creatine clearance, the dose in these cases being 25mg once a day. Other wise the dose is 50 to 100 mg once a day for atenolol. Dosage of Metoprolol is to be individualised which can be 100 to 200mg once a day. The drugs are contraindicated in heart block, sinus bradycardia and cardiac failure. The dosage are to be adjusted in veriant angina, hepatic and renal dysfunction. The drugs should not be withdrawn abruptly.

Betaxolol

This drug is structurally related to metoprolol and is a selective beta one antagonist. Betaxolol hydrochloride also reduces intraocular pressure like timolol. 0.5 percent solution is used for reduction of intraocular pressure for control of chronic open angle glaucoma and ocular hypertension by topical application to the eye. It probably produces its effect by reducing formation of aqueous humor or blocking the endogenous catecholamines which increases the cyclic AMP within the ciliary processes and subsequent formation of aqueous humor. Betaxolol is safe for treating chronic open angle glaucoma in patients with asthma, bronchitis and obstructive pulmonary disease. It is to be used with precaution in cardiac failure, thyrotoxicosis, diabetes melitus and nursing women. Betaxolol may mask the symptoms of thyrotoxicosis and hypoglycaemia. The dose of betaxolol in the treatment of open angle glaucoms or ocular hypertension is one drop of 0.5 percent solution in the affected eye twice daily.

Labetolol

This is a non selective beta blocker with also alpha adrenergic blocking activity. It is used in mild to severe hypertension in a dose of 50mg twice a day. However the dose can be increased upto 600mg twice a day. Labetolol reduces the peripheral vascular resistance without causing reflex tachycardia.

Adverse effects : Labetolol may cause postural hypotension. It is reported to cause jaundice in addition to common side effects of the beta blockers.

Pindolol

Pindolol and Acebutolol are the two non selective beta blockers with intrinsic alpha adrenergic activity. The usual therapeutic dose is 200mg twice a day. Both the drugs may cause myalgia, arthralgia and arthritis in addition to side effects of other beta blockers.

3.9. CENTRALLY ACTING SYMPATHOLYTIC ANTI HYPERTENSIVE AGENTS

These drugs are thought to stimulate the central alfa adrenergic receptors. Stimulation of these presynaptic alfa two receptors situated in the vasomotor center of the brain results in decreased sympathetic tone of the peripheral blood vessels. Clonidine and Methyldopa are the two prototype drugs that act centrally and are predominantly alfa$_2$ receptor agonists.

Clonidine

This drug on intravenous injection causes an initial increase in both systolic and diastolic pressure but on oral administration it does not produce the hypertensive effect. The initial rise in pressure after I.V. administration is seen because it is a partial agonist. This effect is short lived and is soon followed by a fall in blood pressure with decreased cardiac output and heart rate. Clonidine decreases plasma renin activity which is thought to be mediated centrally by decreasing the sympathetic stimulation of the juxtaglomerular cells of the kidney. So the renal vascular resistance decreases although the renal blood flow remains unchanged. The oral dose of the drugs is between 0.1 to 0.8 mg a day. After oral administration within 30 to 60 minutes the peak concentration is obtained and it lasts for about 8 hours. The drug is metabolised and excreted primarily in the urine.

It is used as a single drug or in combination with other antihypertensives in the treatment of moderate to severe hypertension.

Drug interactions : It may enhance the CNS depressant effects of alcohol and sedatives. Tricyclic antidepressants and beta blockers block its antihypertensive effect.

Adverse effects : Dry mouth is a common problem which can be minimized by giving two unequal doses, the larger one being given at bed time. The other side effects are drowsiness, fluid or electrolyte imbalance, orthostatic hypotension, myalgia and impotence.

Methyldopa

This drug is an inhibitor of dopa decarboxylase. Alfa methyl dopa is metabolised by decarboxylation and hydroxylation in the adrenergic neuron of the CNS. The metabolite alfa methyl noradrenaline so formed stimulates the central alfa adrenergic receptors thereby inhibiting the sympathetic tone. Methyl dopa also reduces renal vascular resistance because the metabolite alfa methylnorepinephrine exerts a direct effect on peripheral adrenergic neuron that may also contribute to its anti-hypertensive action. The net effect of methyldopa is reduction of peripheral arteriolar resistance with little effect on cardiac output, renal blood flow or glomerular filtration rate. Methyldopa is given in doses of 500mg to3gm a day in divided doses for control of hypertension. Methyldopa is well absorbed following oral administration and is subjected to first pass metabolism. Peak effect is seen within 4 to 6 hours after its administration and lasts for 24 hours. Methyl-dopa is mainly excereted by the kidneys.

Drug interactions : Beta blockers, general anesthetics and thiazide diuretics are known to increase the hypotensive effect of methyldopa, therefore dose reduction may be required when concomitantly used. Methyldopa increases the pressor effects of noradrenaline and other sympathomimetics.

Adverse reactions : Sedation is common side effect of methyldopa which may decrease with continued use. It may produce drug fever accompained by alteration in liver function, oedema, weight gain, bradycardia and haemolytic anaemia. The other adverse effects are impotence, gastrointestinal disorders, salivary gland inflammation, breast enlargement, myalgia, rash, thrombocytopenia and granulomatous skin eruption.

3.10. POST GANGLIONIC ADRENERGIC NEURON BLOCKERS

These drugs are selective inhibitors of sympathetic neuronal function by virtue of interference with chemical mediation at the adrenergic ganglionic nerve endings involvng one or more mechanisms.

Guanethidine

This drug is used in the teatment of severe hypertension usually in combination with a diuretic and a vasodilator. Guanethidine acts presynaptically to inhibit the release of the neurotransmitter from peripheral adrenergic neurons thus reducing the response of the sympathetic nerve activation. Guanethidine is taken up and stored at the adrenergic nerve ending in a manner similar to noradrenaline uptake and storage. Guanethidine does not cross the blood brain barrier so it does not effect the noradrenaline stores in the CNS. It also reduces the plasma renin activity. It causes bradycardia because it depresses vasoconstrictor reflexes, so postural hypotension is commonly encountered. Guanethedine is given in a dose of 5 to 10 mg a day. The absorption of the drug varies in different individuals. It can be from 3 to 30 percent of the dose, however it has a long duration of action. The drug is metabolised by the liver and is excreted in the urine.

Drug interactions and adverse effects : Many agents that prevent the uptake of guanethidine in the nerve terminal block the drug's antihypertensive effect, eg tricyclic antidepressant like amitriptyline inhibits the effects of guanethedine in this manner. It is contraindicated with MAO inhibitors like isocarboxazide, tranylcypromine and phenelzine. The drug has direct inhibtory effect on skeletal muscle contraction and can cause muscular weakness. The other side effects are orthostatic hypotension and salt and water retention. Parasympathetic predominance following sympathetic blockade results in gastrointestinal hyperactivity inducing diarrhea.

3.11. RENIN ANGIOTENSIN ANTAGONIST

Renin, a proteolytic enzyme is synthesized, stored and secreted by the juxtaglomerular cells of the kidney. It plays important role in regulation of blood pressure by catalyzing the conversion of angiotensinogen to angiotensin I. Thereafter an enzyme peptidyl dipeptidase converts angiotensin I to angiotensin II which is a potent vasoconstrictor. Drugs that interfere with renin-angiotensin system are represented by Captopril, Enalapril and Lisinopril. These drugs produce their antihypertensive effect by interfering either with the formation or utilization of angiotensin II and thereby reducing the vasoconstrictor effect.

Captopril

This drug is a specific inhibitor of angiotensin converting enzyme (ACE) peptidyl dipeptidase and therefore it inhibits vasoconstriction. It also inhibits sodium and water retention because of less aldosterone secretion which is the promoter of sodium and water retention in the body. Captopril may also increase the concentration of bradykinin in the body which is a potent vasodilator.

An average dose of 75 to 100 mg per day is used in the treatment of mild to modrate hypertension. Captopril causes a total reduction of peripheral resistance reflected by a fall in mean arterial blood pressure and either no change or an increase in cardiac output. Captopril is effective in relieving chronic congestive heart failure by reducing preload and afterload. Captopril is rapidly absorbed following oral administration, the onset of action is seen within two hours of administration. 95 percent of the drug is eliminated by the kidneys within 24 hours.

Drug interactions and adverse effects : Severe hypotension with initial dose in patients on diuretic therapy. Increased potassium levels with concurrent use of potassium sparing diuretics. It can cause proteinurea. Mnitoring urinary protein level is therefore recommended with the treatment. Captopril is contraindicated in patients with bilateral renal artery stenosis. Skin rash is reported in 10 percent cases.

Enalapril

This drug is also an ACE inhibitor having similar pharmacological actions as that of Captopril. Enalapril is a prodrug which is converted in the body to Enalaprilate which is more potent with a longer duration of action. Older patients above the age of 65 yrs require only 5mg daily. In renal impairement the dose is 2.5 mg daily. In others the maximum daily dose is 40mg.

Drug interactions and adverse effects : Potassium sparing diuretics induce hyperkalaemia. Other diuretics enhance anti-hypertensive effects. Enalapril may increase the lithium blood level in patients on lithium carbonate. Initial hypotension with enalopril may be severe and prolonged. The other reactions are dizziness headache, fatigue, cough, lassitude, rash, and renal failure. It is contraindicated in pregnancy.

Lisinopril

This is a synthetic peptide derivative, orally acting ACE inhibitor with longer duration of action. Supression of the renin-angiotensin-aldosterone axis lowers the blood pressure.

Peak serum concentration occurs in 7 hours after oral administration. It is not bound to the plasma proteins. It is not metabolised and excreted entirely in the urine in the unchanged form. Multiple dosing exhibits half life to be about 12 hours. Impaired renal function decreases its excretion. Onset of action is after one hour of administration and anti-hypertensive effect is observed for 24 hours. The dose of the drug is 2.5 mg once a day. Maximum dose can be upto 20mg a day.

Drug interactions and adverse effects : Concomitant administration of hydrochlorthiazide produces further reduction of blood pressure. Indomethacin reduces the anti-hypertensive effects. Abrupt withdrawal can cause rebound hypertension. Adverse effects are dizziness, diarrhoea and respiratory symptoms with cough.

3.12. CATECHOLAMINE DEPLETERS FROM THE ADRENERGIC NERVE TERMINALS

Rauwolfia alkaloids can be used in the treatment of hypertension, however they are not used commonly because of their large number of adverse effects. Reserpine the rauwoifia alkaloid is used in combination with other drugs in a dose of 0.1mg two to three times a day. Reserpine produces its effect through depletion of the stores of catechol-amines from the adrenergic neurones. It also inhibits the uptake of noradrenaline into the vesicles of the nerve terminal. Intraneuronal degradation of noradrenaline also occurs both centrally and peripherally. Oral administration of reserpine takes a long time to produce antihypertensive effect because of the time factor involved in the depletion of the catecholamine stores.

Drug interactions and adverse effects : Hypotensive effects are enhanced by the thiazide diuretics and beta blockers. Reserpine increases cardiac glycoside toxicity. Tricyclic antidepressants antagonise the effect of reserpine. Reserpine has a number of adverse effects, the prominent one being sedation owing to the depleted stores of catecholamines and 5 - hydroxytryptamine of the brain. It may cause psychic depression that may result in suicidal tendency. The other side effects are gastric ulceration abdominal cramp and diarrhoea, nasal congestion and occasional extrapyramidal reactions.

3.13. ALFA ADRENERGIC BLOCKING AGENTS

These drugs bind to the peripheral adrengergic receptors thereby blocking the pressure effects of sympathomimetic amines. Of haloalkyal amine derivatives phenoxybenzamine, phentolamine (Regitine), Tolazoline are the representative drugs.

Phenoxybenzamine

This drug has limited use in the management of pheochromocytoma and hypertension before surgery. The dose of the drug varies from 20 to 60mg. Though it is orally effective it is given as injection because of its gastric irritant properties.

Phentolamine (regitine)

Phentolamine is used parenterally in a dose of 5mg having the same indication as phenoxybenzamine.

Tolazoline (priscoline)

This alfa adrenergic blocker is used in a dose of 10 to 50mg four times a day. The drug is absorbed from both oral and parentral route. However oral route is less effective because tolazoline is rapidly excreted in the urine.

Adverse effects : All these drugs have common side effects. They produce reflex tachycardia, postural hypotension; nasal stuffiness and gastrointestinal stimulation.

3.14. ARTERIAL AND VENOUS VASODILATORS

These drugs reduce the arterial resistance and venous tone thereby reducing the blood pressure. The prototype drugs of this group are Diazoxide, Sodium nitroprusside, prazosine, Hydralazine.

Diazoxide

This is a non diuretic analogue of thiazide. It has the capacity to relax arteriolar smooth muscles directly with out any action on the venous capacitance. This drug is indicated in hypertensive emergencies and is administered intravenously in a dose of 5mg/kg body weight, repeated every 6 to 8 hours up to a total dose of 300 to 1200 mg a day. Diazoxide gets bound to plasma protein rapidly and half life is about 60 hours. The drug is metabolized by the liver and one third of it is excreted in the urine unchanged. *Adverse effects and contraindications*. Diazoxide can cause fluid retention if it is used for more than 24 hours. It is contra-indicated in angina and myocardial infarction.

Sodium Nitroprusside

This agent acts directly on the arterial and venous smooth muscles without having effect on other smooth muscles. Sodium nitroprusside increases the venous capacitance and results in decreased cardiac preload and so decreases myocardial oxygen demand. Renal blood flow is maintained, however the drug is inactivated rapidly by the hepatic enzymes. Therefore, it is administered as intravenous infusion with five percent dextrose solution. Nitroprusside decomposes in light so the preparation is to be protected from light. Nitroprusside is used for hypertensive emergencies and is preferred over diazoxide in patients with coronary insufficiency or in pulmonary edema. The drug is also beneficial in the treatment of acute congestive heart failure. It lowers the ventricular filling pressure and thus can improve ventricular function in patients with acute myocardial infarction.

Adverse effects : The untoward effects of nitroprusside are hypotension and that is why blood pressure is to be monitored while the drug is administered. The other effects are palpitation and nausea. Prolonged nitroprusside therapy with poor renal function can cause muscle spasm with weakness. Nitropruside can interfere with iodine transport so it can cause hypothyroidism.

Hydralazine

Hydralazine produces its effect by direct relaxation of the arteriolar smooth muscles to produce vasodilation. It reduces the diastolic pressure more than systolic blood pressure. The usual dose of the drug is 25 to 100 mg in a day, however the dose is to be adjusted in elderly patients and in renal function impairment. It is well absorbed from the oral route and the peak blood concentration is obtained within half hour to two hours of the oral administration. Hydralazine is metabolised by the liver through many pathways of which acetylation is the main pathway. The process of acetylation is under genetic control so slow acetylators can give rise to a higher plasma concentration than the fast acetylators for the same concentration of the drug. 85 percent of the drug is bound to the plasma proteins.

Besides oral administration the drug can be given parenterally for a quick effect which is seen within 10 to 20 minutes and lasts for 2 to 4 hours.

Drug interaction and adverse effects : Antihypertensive effects of hydralazine is enhanced by MAO inhibitors, tricyclic antidepressants and diuretics of thiazide group. Tachycardia is the common side effect which is counteracted by beta blockers. The other side effects are dizziness and palpitation, severe headache, anorexia vomiting. Hydralazine causes fluid retention which can be counteracted by the use of diuretics.

Prazosin

Prazosin is a quinazoline derivative. It blocks the post synaptic alfa receptors of the blood vessels thereby causing vasodilation of the arteries and veins. It produces a minimal change in the cardiac output, renal blood flow and the glomerular filtration rate.

Large extent of the durg gets protein bound and the plasma half life lies between 2 to 3 hours. It is used in the treatment of moderate hypertension in a dose of 1 mg a day along with a diuretic.

Drug interactions and adverse effects : Prazosin effect is potentiated with other anti hypertensives and diuretics so hypotension with sudden loss of consciousness can be seen in sodium depleted individuals who are on other anti hypertensive drugs. In congestive heart failure the plasma half life can be prolonged which can cause hypotension and syncope due to decreased venous return to the heart. Other side effects are dry mouth, nasal stuffiness, lassitude and constipation.

4

DRUGS ACTING ON THE CENTRAL NERVOUS SYSTEM

The central nervous system (CNS) comprises of the brain and the spinal cord. Drugs acting on the CNS are believed to alter the cellular functioning of the nerve cells or the transmission of impulse between the nerve cells which involves a chemical neurotransmitter. Drugs interact with the neurotransmitter at a specific site in the CNS.

These drugs can be classified according to their therapeutic use as follows :

- (a) Hypnotics and sedatives
- (b) Anxiolytics and tranquillizers
- (c) Antipsychotics, anti depressants and mood elevators.
- (d) General anaesthetics
- (e) Anti epileptics
- (f) Antiparkinsonism drugs
- (g) Narcotic analgesics
- (h) CNS stimulants

4.1. BARBITURATES

Barbiturates are the representative group of agents that are used as sedative hypnotics. Barbituric acid derivatives depress the CNS at all levels in a dose dependent manner which is the basis for their use as sedative and hypnotics.

4.1.1. The classification of Barbiturates

Barbiturates can be classified according to their onset and duration of action. These properties are dependent on their rate of metabolic degradation, lipid solubility and extent of protein binding since this reduces its renal excretion.

I. Long acting barbiturates, e.g. phenobarbital and barbital. They are effective for more than 6 hours as sedative and hypnotic.

At a low dose they are used as antiepileptic. The antieplleptic dose of phenobarbital is 30 mg three times a day.

The drug is long acting because of slow oxidation in liver. Phenobarbital is also capable of inducing the liver microsomal drug metabolizing enzyme system with increased degradation of the barbiturates leading to barbiturate tolerance. There is also increased inactivation of many drugs such as anticoagulants, phenytoin, digitoxin, theophyllin and glucocorticoids which lead to drug interactions when prescribed together.

II. Ultra short acting e.g. Thiopental acts within seconds of its administration with the duration of action of about 30 minutes. It is used as an intravenous anesthetic agent.

The ability of any agent to affect the CNS is dependent on its ability to cross blood brain barrier. Blood brain barrier is constituted by the lining of the brain capillaries and the foot processes of astrocytes. These capillaries unlike those in other tissues have some pinocytic vesicles. Lipid soluble substances remain unionized at physiological pH and are poorly bound to plasma proteins and therefore are able to diffuse across the blood-brain barrier. The ultra short acting barbiturates due to their high lipid solubility reach the brain tissue and get redistributed to the other tissues e.g. the muscle, in a very short time. So they have a very short duration of action since they remain in the CNS for a very short time.

III. Short acting barbiturates are represented by Pentobarbital, Hexobarbital and Secobarbital. They have about 2 hours duration of action and their chief use is in sleep induction.

IV. Intermediate acting barbiturates are those which have effect for about 3 to 5 hours. The examples are Amobarbital and Butobarbital which are used as hypnotics. They produce hangover effect because of residual depression of CNS.

4.1.2. Mechanism of action of Barbiturates

Barbiturares have gama aminobutyric acid (GABA) like action or enhance the effect of GABA which is an inhibitory neurotransmitter. Barbiturates may also inhibit the neuronal uptake of GABA or may stimulate its release. At higher dose barbiturates produce generalised depression of CNS with respiratory depression.

Other pharmacological actions : The ability of barbiturates to stimulate liver glucuronyl transferase has been applied in the treatment of hyperbilirubinemia in neonates. Barbiturates do not have analgesic properties. At sedative dose they have little effect on the cardiovascular system. However at increased dose depression of ganglionic transmission occurs with fall in blood pressure and heart rate.

4.1.3. Toxic effects of barbiturates

At toxic dose circulatory collapse occurs due to medullary and vasomoter depression. At anesthetic dose barbiturtes can supress renal tubular transport. Barbiturates can induce porphyria due to the disturbance in porphyrin metabolism characterised by increased formation and excretion of porphyrins which are fundamental ring structure of heamoglobin.

Barbiturates produce physiologic and psychologic dependence. Withdrawl of the drug can result in seizures, tremor and hallucination. Treatment of barbiturate poisoning consists of supporting respiration and circulation. Excretion of the drug is enhanced by alkalinizing the urine and promoting diuresis. Haemodialysis and peritoneal dialysis is required in acute over dosage.

4.2. NON BARBITURRATE SEDATIVE HYPNOTICS

The drugs belonging to this group are Chloral hydrate, paraldehyde, Methyprolone. Chloral hydrate a is safe hypnotic which induces sleep for 6 hours. It causes bad taste and gastrointestinal irritation and so it finds limited use. The CNS depression is potentiated by alcoholic drinks. The dose of the drug is 300 mg.

Paraldehyde produces quick hypnotic effect which lasts for 4 to 8 hours. It is mainly used in patients undergoing treatment of withdrwal from alcohol. It is administered rectally as retention anema by diluting in suitable vegetable oil in a 1:2 ratio. The dose is between 2 to 8 ml.

Methapyrolone although a non barbiturate resembles secobarbital in its action with very limited therapeutic use.

4.3. ANXIOLYTICS, TRANQUILLISERS.

Benzodiazepine and their derivatives like lorazepam, flurazepam, chlordiazepoxide, diazepam are used as anxiolytics. Benzodiazepines are not general neuronal depressants which makes them different from barbiturate group of sedatives. These group of drugs are absorbed rapidly from the gastrointestinal tract. The elimination half life varies from agent to agent. Benzodiazepines can be grouped according to their elimination half life.

   I. Triazolam and Loprazolam have very short half life up to 4 hours.

   II. Lormetazepam, Temezepam, and Zopiclone have short half life which varies from 4 to 12 hours.

   III. Intermediate half life is shown by Lorazepam and Oxazepam which range from 12 to 20 hours.

   IV. Long half life which can be more than 20 hours e.g. Nitrazepan fluzepam and diazepam. Diazepam as such has short half life but its metabolites are active with a longer half life, therefore, it becoms long acting when given over a long period. Pharmacological effects of benzodiazepines are shown because they act by binding to specific benzodiazepine receptors which help to potentiate the binding of GABA. In animal experiments benzodiazepine has been shown to prevent strychnine induced convulsion. Because they increase seizure threshold they are useful in status epilepticus. They have minimal effect on cardiovascular system so they are useful as sedative and anxiolytics. The usual dose of diazepam for anxiety tension is 2 to 10 mg. per day in divided doses. Other specific use of benzodiazepines are in preanesthetic medication and treatment of alcohol withdrawal syndromes. The unwanted effects of benzodiazepines are ataxia and potentiation of other CNS depressants like alcohol and barbiturates.

4.4. ANTIPSYCHOTICS

These group of drugs are used in the treatment of illness that is characterised by change in personality with disintregrated and detachment from social environment. The cardinal features are disorder of thinking with incoherent disjointed emotion.

Phenothiazines and Butyrophenones

Both the drugs produce improvement of mood and behavior without excessive sedation. Phenothiazine dreivatives are *Chlorpromazine, Fluphenazine, Triflupromazine* and Thioridazine used as antipsychotics. Mode of action of these drugs are because of their antidopaminergic activity in the limbic nigrostriatal and hypothalamic system because dopamine is one of the neurotransmitters involved in this system.

This antagonism produces emotional quietening and reduction of physical activity. Most phenothiazines are anti-emetic, in animal experiments apomorphine (CTZ stimulant) induced vomiting is antagonized. At higher dose they may be direct depressant of medullary vomiting center. Phenothiazine derivatives produce hypothermia, depress hypothalamic function which control and intergrate the peripheral autonomic mechanism, endocrine activity and somatic function. Endocrine functional change bring about release of prolactin inducing lactation, gynecomastia, decrease in corticotropin release, secretion of pituitary growth bormone leading to weight gain and increase in appetite. The dose of chlorpromazine is 25 mg three times a day and Fluphenazine Img a day in anxiety and tension.

Side effects of Chlorpromazine : All chlorpromazine group of drugs show extrapyramidal side effects such as parkinsonian rigidity and tremors because it is a dopamine antagonist in the basal ganglia. Phenothiazine causes orthostatic hypotension due to its alpha adrenergic blocking action. Besides the anti psychotic action some phenothiazine derivatives show anti cholinergic and anti histaminic effect. Phenothiazine potentiates the action of alcohol and barbiturates.

The other antipsychotic drugs are Butyrophenone and Thioxanthine derivatives, viz. *Chlorprothixine* and *Thiothixine* both the drugs having similar pharmacological effects as that of phenothiazine. *Haloperidol* and *droperidol* are the prototype butyrophenones resembling phenothiazines in their pharmacological actions and side effects. The dose of haloperidol is 1.5 to 2mg. a day.

Lithium carbonate is the inorganic salt effective in controlling manic depressive state. The daily dose is 800 to 1600 mg. Since lithium carbonate has a low therapeutic index serum concentration has to be between 0.8 to 1.5 meq. per liter of the blood accordingly the dose is determined. Lithium is well absorbed from the gastrointestinal tract and is eliminated in urine, however 80% of lithium is reabsorbed in the proximal tubule. Lithium may produce its pharmacological effect by stabilization of dopamineric receptor through inactivation of hormone sensitive adenylate cyclase. Side effects of lithium are anorexia, vomiting, thirst.

Toxic effects include hypotension, cardiac arrhythmias and enlargment of thyroid gland. Intoxication with lithium can be reversed by osmotic diuretic like manitol.

4.5. MOOD ELEVATORS

There are two principal groups of antidepressants used in depressive illness. They are tricyclic drugs like *Imipramine*, *Amitriptyline* and *Trimipramine* all of which are catechol amine reuptake inhibitors. The other group consists of *monamine oxidase (MAO) inhibitors e.g. phenelzine, Isocarboxazide, tranylcypromine* and *Mebenazine*.

Amitriptyline is better tolerated than imipramine and is chemically related to phenothiazine. Tricyclic antidepressants potentiate the effect of catecholamines by blocking the reuptake of biogenic amines after presynaptic release. They produce their effect as mood elevator in 2 to 3 weeks of administration. The dose of amitriptyline is 25 mg. 3 to 4 times a day.

The side effects of these drugs are orthostatic hypotension, anticholinergic effects and dizziness with muscle tremor.

MAO inhibitors : The two effective drugs of this group viz. Phenelzine and Isocarboxazide prevent oxidative deamination of the bigoenic amines noradrenaline, tyramine and dopamine. They produce an increase of biogenic amines in brain thereby poducing their antidepressant effect. Isocarboxazide and

Phenelzine is used in a dose of 10 to 30 mg and 15 to 30mg a day respectively. Side effects are hypotension by affecting the ganglionic transmission. They interact with tyramine containing food like cheese. The unmetabolised tyramine can produce hypertensive crisis. It also potentiate ephedrines and tricyclic antidepressants. These drugs are contraindicated in liver disease, congestive heart failure and epilepsy.

4.6. GENERAL ANAESTHETICS

Anaesthesia denotes loss of feeling and insensibility which can be general or local. Anaesthetics are group of agents that produce this loss of feeling and insensibility and are used in surgical procedures. They can be gaseous anaesthetics such as ether, halothane, enflurane, isoflurane, nitrous oxide or intravenous anaesthetic such as thiopental sodium and methohexitone. The ultra short acting barbituretes are used for the induction of gaseous anaesthetics. Ketamine, a non barbiturate is used in a dose of I to 2mg. body weight for the same purpose. However the drug can not be used in hypertension, psychiatric disorders and in increased intraocular pressure.

Pharmacological Actions of General Anaesthetics

Aneasthetic agents should have smooth induction and produce adequate muscle relaxation without respiratory depression. However, all general anaesthetics depress all parts of the CNS with considerable regional differences and the phenomenon is dose dependent. The higher cortical centers and the ascending reticular activiating system are most susceptible to the general anaesthetics and are affected at a lower concentration. But when the anaesthetic concentration in the brain increases it depresses the lower centers leading to respiratory and circulatory failure.

As the drugs are administered by inhalation the concentration of the anaesthetic agents in blood is kept under control at a desired level which determines the various stages and planes of anaesthesia. The stages of anesthesia are recognised from changes in respiration rate and pattern, muscle tone and reflex action specially that of eyes. Anaesthetics produce different effects on the autonomic nervous system.

Diethyl ether and cyclopropane are sympathetic stimulants. On the other hand halothane causes inhibition of the sympathetic nervous system. At a higher blood level all general anaesthetics depress the respiratory system.

Anaesthetics produce dose related negative inotropic effect on the heart. However different anaesthetics differ quantitatively in this respect. e.g., halothane depresses the myocardium more than ether. The overall effect on the myocardium and the depression of the peripheral circulation producing fall in blood pressure is dose dependent. Anaesthetics have different hepatic and metabolic action. They are metabolized to various degrees depending upon their structure and partition coefficient eg. methoxy flurane has greater metabolism. 50% of the agent is absorbed and metabolized to free fluoride ion which can cause renal damage.

4.6.1. Preanaesthetic Medication

Several drugs are used prior to induction of anaesthesia. The object of such medication is to sedate and produce anxiety free state for the smooth induction of anaesthesia and reduce the side effects of the anaesthetic agents. In additon drugs are administered to decrease vagal tone and block bronchial and other secretions.

1. Muscarinic blockers, Atropine sulphate and Hyoscine hydrobromide are given to block the side effects of irritant anaesthetics like diethyl ether and cyclopropane.
2. Narcotic analgesics, Morphine, Meperidine or Fentanyl group of drugs are administered to reduce anxiety. However they can potentiate the respiratory depression of anaesthetics which they themselves possess.
3. Anxiolytic and Sedatives like diazepam and short acting barbiturates are administered to diminish anxiety and produce drowsy state which helps in smooth induction of anaesthesia.

4.7. ANTI EPILEPTIC DRUGS

Epileptic convulsions or fit is the disorder of cerebral function accompanied by sudden excessive electrical discharge from cerebral neurones. The electrical activity can be recorded by electroencephalogram (EEG). The discharge of the abnormal group of cells is goverened by the balance at a given time between two opposing factors. Acetylcholine is an excitatory transmitter and gama aminobutyric acid (Gaba) is an inhibitory transmitter. So GABA agonist or drugs having GABA like action or which enhance the effect of GABA e.g. barbiturates or benzodiazepines form the core drug for the control of epileptic fits. Phenytoin, phenobarbitone, pirimidone and carbamazepine are the effective drugs used in the treatment of grandmal epilepsy which is a generalised seizure with loss of consciousness. They are effective in focal epilepsy due to discharge arising in localised area of the cortex e.g. in Jacksonian march.

Phenytoin

Chemically this is diphenyl hydantoin, It exerts its dampening effect only when neuronal activity is abnormally high. It allows normal conduction of action potentials but stops the seizures.

Being a weak acid the intestinal absorption of phenytoin is variable and 90% of it is plasma protein bound. It is excreted in bile and urine after microsomal metabolism. Hepatic metabolism of this drug varies because of genetic abnormalities. So the blood level should be monitored, the average daily dose is between 200 to 400mg. Since it has a half life greater than 24 hours it can be given once a day. The dose is tailored to the individual need and response. Phenytoin may be given in combination with phenobarbitone or carbamazepine. But serum level of phenytoin is reduced because of induction of hepatic enzyme when given in combination with carbamazepine.

Phenytoin is contraindicated in petitmal epilepsy. Petitmal is a type of attack with transient loss of consciousness that may last for 10 to 15 seconds which may be accompained by myoclonic jerking of arms. Petitmal may start in childhood. The other side effects are drowsiness, osteomalacia and folate deficiency resulting in megaloblastic anaemia and gingival hyperplasia in children.

Drug Interaction : If concurrently administered with chloramphenicol, isonazid, dicumarol and sulphonamides increase of phenytoin concentration in blood is observed because of inactivation of metabolising enzymes.

Ethosuximide

This is the most useful drug in the treatment of petitmal epilepsy. The other drugs belonging to this group are methosuximide and fensuximide. Ethosuximide is effective in a dose of 750 to 1500 mg daily. It is well absorbed from the gastrointestinal tract, 80% of the dose is metabolized and 20% is excreted unchanged in the urine with the other metabolites. Untoward effects are gastrointestinal reactions and anorexia, nausea. Drowsiness, headache photophobia and extrapyramidal symptoms have also been reported.

Primodone

The drug is useful in both grandmal and partial seizures. The drug is well absorbed on oral administration in a dose of 125 to 500 mg a day. One of the major metabolites is phenobarbitone, so it is not given in combination with phenobarbitone. Initially primodone produces sedation but this effect decreases with continued use. Pyrimidone is contraindicated in petitmal epilepsy.

Sodium Valproate

This drug differs in chemical structure from other antiepileptics. It is effective in a dose of 600 to 2600 mg. in divided doses to be given after meals. It acts by inhibiting enzymatic break down of GABA which is carried out by GABA transaminase and thus terminates fits.

The drug is teratogenic and can cause pancreatitis and hepatic failure specially when given in combination with other antiepileptics. Anorexia, nausea, ataxia are the other side effects. It produces drug interaction with phenobarbitone by causing a 40% rise in the blood level of phenobarbitone.

Carbamazepine

This drug is used in a dose of 200mg once or twice initially which can be increased to 400mg two to three times a day in the treatment of grandmal epilepsy. Anticonvulsant effect is similar to that of phenytoin. The untoward effects are ataxia, nausea, atropine like effect and bone marrow depression kindey and liver toxicity have also been reported.

4.8. DRUGS USED IN THE TREATMENT OF PARKINSONISM

Parkinson's disease can also be termed as Parkinsonian syndrome in which there is muscular rigidity and tremor associated with cellular loss and pigmentation of substantia niagra. However, many drugs notably those of phenothiazine group, reserpine, butyrophenone may induce Parkinsonism as a side effect which is referred as extrapyramidal effect. Drug induced Parkinsonism is curable if the drug is discontinued.

In majority of parkinsonian patients the cause of the syndrome is not known and treatment is designed to ameliorate the disability. The most general effective therapy is a combination of anticholinergic drug with levodopa and dopa decarboxylase inhibitor. Dopamine deficiency in the striatum needs to be corrected in Parkinsonism. As dopamine cannot cross the blood brain barrier, levodopa the precursor of dopamine is administered.

Levodopa

500 mg tablets are available, the dose of the drug is between 1 gm to 8 gm daily in divided doses. Effects of levodopa are enhanced by the peripheral dopa decarboxylase inhibitors like carbidopa. More than 90 percent of orally ingested levodopa is metabolized in the extra cerebral tissue so it does not reach the target site in the brain. If the drug is given with the dopa decarboxylase inhibitor, carbidopa, then selective inhibition of the extra cerebral dopa decarboxylase reduces the amount of levodopa required to show a therapeutic effect. This combination reduces the side effect of levodopa like nausea, vomiting and cardiac arrythmias. Combination of levodopa and dopadecarboxylase inhibitor is available in tablets containing 100mg of levodopa and 25 mg of carbidopa. The recomended dose is one tablet 3-4 times a day up to maximum of 8 tablets per day. Drug interactions of levodopa are numerous. Pyridoxine reduces the benificial effect of levodopa; phenothiazine derivatives and butyrophenon antagonize the effect of levodopa; MAO inhibitors such as isocarboxazide, iproniazide which are used as antidepressant are contraindicated in patients taking levodopa.

Anticholinergic agents produce synergistic effect with levodopa. Anticholinergic drugs produce modest improvement in the early course of the disease. There are several synthetic drugs viz.

(a) Benhexol hydrochloride, dose 2 or 5 mg.

(b) Benztropin, dose 2 mg.

(c) Orphanadrine, 30mg.

Any one of these drugs is introduced in small amounts, one tablet of the above streingth can be given twice daily. The common adverse effects of anticholinergic drugs like dry mouth or blurring of vision are encountered. The dose is to be reduced to minimize these side effects. The initiation of antiparkinsonian treatment with a combination of orally active dopamine receptor agonist bromocriptine and a small dose of levodopa can also be useful.

Bromocriptine

Bromocriptine is an ergot derivative which mimics all the actions of dopamine. The initial dose is 2.5 mg twice daily which is gradually built up to 30 to 40 mg daily. It can be given alone or with levodopa. The drug shows the untoward effect of hallucination and hypotension. The other adverse effects are dizziness, nasal congestion, depression and ataxia.

Drug interactions

Potentiation of antihypertensive effect requires dose adjustment. Psychotropic drugs are to be avoided.

Amantadine

It stimulates the release of dopamine from dopaminergic nerve endings and delays its reuptake. Amantadine is absorbed from the oral route and is excreted unchanged in urine. Amantadine may be more effective than anticholinergics in parkinsonism. However the drug induces tolerance after use for some time.

4.9. NORCOTIC ANALGESICS

Analgesics are used for the relief of pain. They are of two types viz. narcotic analgesic and non narcotic analgesics.

Narcotic analgesics : These consist of opium alkaloids and their derivatives. Morphine, the principal alkaloid in opium and related opiates are used therapeutically to relieve pain in myocardial infarction, surgery, terminal illness and obstetrical manipulation. To produce analgesic effect and other pharmacological actions the prime requirement for morphine and related opioids is binding at the opioid receptors. Opioid receptors are of many types which are located within the CNS.

The sites are the limbic system, amygdaloid nucleus and hypothalamus which are associated with autonomic function and certain aspect of emotion and behavior. The other sites are the chemoreceptor trigger zone (CTZ), which is in control of nausea and vomiting and the nucleus of solitary tract which is the location of cough center. Thus from the distribution of opioid receptor it is obvious that morphine which produces its effect by binding to these opioid receptors will either produce agonistic or antagonistic effect on the physiological processes connected with the above sites of stimulation.

Endogenous opioids : Two naturally occuring peptides have been isolated from the brain that are associated with pain and analgesia.

4.9.1. Enkephalin

These are naturally occuring penta peptides isolated from the brain that have potent opiate like effect and probably serve as neurotransmitter of the endogenous opioid. Neurons containing enkephalins are widely distributed in the CNS that are involved in the transmission of pain.

Endorphin : Endorphins are a group of endogenous polypeptide brain substances that bind to opiate receptors in the various areas of the brain and thereby raise pain threshold. The role of endorphins can be assessed by the effect of antagonist of the opiates, e.g. naloxone. Such agents block the effect of endogenously secreted opiate peptides.

4.9.2. Morphine

It is an alkaloid isolated from opium. Its CNS effects are analgesia with increased tolerance to pain, euphoria, mental clouding with out loss of consciousness. Morphine can produce nausea and vomiting as it stimulates the CTZ.

The other pharmacological effects are dose dependent respiratory depression. It produces miosis and pin point pupil which is an indication of acute toxicity. Morphine and its derivatives are potent cough suppresant. Morphine produces depression of vasomotor medullary center, it also releases histamine so orthostatic hypotension can occur. The release of histamine can induce bronchoconstriction and is contraindicated in asthmatics. Morphine reduces peristalsis and results in constipation. Morphine is absorbed from the oral route but the preferred route is intra muscular injection. 90% of the given dose is excreted in the urine and 10% in the feaces as conjugated morphine. Metabolism occurs in the liver. Average adult dose for analgesia is 10mg intramuscularly. It is used for the control of severe cardiac pain and renal colic. The chief unwanted effect of morphine is that its long term chronic administration results in physical dependence. The other effects are nausea, dysphoria and increase in biliary tract pressure and is therefore contraindicated in gall bladder diseases. Phenothiazines increase the sedative and respiratory depression of morphine group of drugs so their concomitant administration is avoided.

4.9.3. Codeine

The pharmacological effects are very similar to morhine but with lower addiction liability. The action of codeine is much weaker than morphine and does not depress respiration even in large doses. It is used for its cough suppressant action and the antitussive dose is 60mg in divided doses. Codeine is used in cough syrups along with antihistamins and expectorants like ammonium chloride.

Adverse drug reactions of codeine are constipation, nausea, vomiting, dizziness. drowsiness, and dependence.

4.9.4. Pholcodine

This is a derivative of morphine that resembles codeine in suppressing cough. It can be used in children as it does not cause constipation and is less toxic than codeine. It is used in doses of 5 to 15 mg a day.

4.9.5. Methadone

It is a strong analgesic of similar potency to morphine. It is less sedative and euphoritic in its action. However tolerance to analgesic effects and respiratory depressant effect remains the same as morphine.

It is used in the treatment of morphine dependence because withdrawal of the drug has lesser unpleasant effects. The drug is used in a dose of 10mg a day.

4.9.6. Pentazocine

This is a synthetic analgesic with similar action to morphine. Smaller dose of the drug has a more prolonged action. Due to its weak antagonistic effect it can be used in withdrawal of morphine addicts.

Sedation, hallucination, respiratory depression is much less than morphine and tolerance to analgesia is similar to other opioids.

4.10. MORPHINE ANTAGONISTS

N-allyl derivative of oxymorphone i.e. *Naloxone* is considered to be a pure opioid antagonist with no agonistic activity. These group of agents are used to counteract the respiratory depression, sedative effect, and other untoward effects of morphine like drugs. However, on administration of naloxone to addicts of morphine withdrawal symptoms are precipitated and the duration of antagonistic effect remains for 3 to 4 hours. The other agents of this group are *Nalorphin and Naltrexone*. Nalorphin or N-allyl morphine is a partial antagonist. It is used as an antidote for morphine, methadone and pethidine. The side effects of nalorphin is similar to morphine like respiratory depression and fall in blood pressure.

Naltrexone

It is a drug of choice for deaddiction in patients addicted to heroin like opioids. It is a pure antagonist which can be given orally. It is twice as active as naloxone with three times its duration of action. Adverse effects are insomnia, anxiety, abdominal cramps, nausea and joint pain. The drug is contraindicated in hepatic insufficiency.

4.11. ETHYL ALCOHOL AND DRUGS USED IN ALCOHOLISM

Alcohol is not a drug but it is used by man as a beverage from the earliest time. Wines and beers generally contain a low percentage of alcohol. The stronger spirits are prepared by distillation which raises the percentage of alcohol to 30 to 60% and removes the nonvolatile fermentation products of sugar from which most alchohlic liquors are prepared. Alcohol is extensively used as vehicle in pharmaceutical preparations like tinctures and fluid extracts of medicinal agents.

Pharmacological Effects of Alcohol

Local Action

It has irritant action due to its dehydrating property and property of partial precipitation of proteins of the cells. Alcohol in a dilute solution of 25 to 30% strength is used externally as a cooling application on the skin. It is used in preventing bedsoars in a concentration of 50% which hardens the epidermis. A 70% solution is used as an antiseptic application.

Nervous System

Depression of the nervous system is the principal pharmacological action of alcohol . It causes increased secretion of the cerebrospinal fluid and raises the pressure in the subarachnoid space which accounts in part for its ofter effects.

Respiration and Circulation

Effect of alcohol on respiration is inconsistent. The medulla functions even after complete unconsciousness and disappearance of ordinary reflexes.

Effect of alcohol on blood pressure and heart rate is variable. In revere intoxication there is marked reduction in the cerebral circulation and metabolism.

Digestive Tract

Alcohol increases secretion of saliva and gastric secretion which is attributed to the liberation of histamine and gastrin in addtion to the local reflex and psychic effects.

Metabolism : Alcohol dehydrogenase is required for oxidation of alcohol to acetaldehyde which occurs in liver. After absorption, the rate of disappearance or elimination has been worked out to be 100mg per kg per hour. This elimination rate cannot be accelerated by increasing the metabolic rate by administration of drugs or exercise.

In man only 5% of the ingested alcohol is exereted while rest undergoes combustion in the tissue. Alcohol exerts a sparing action of endogenous protein utilization.

Other effects : Alcohol produces tolerance and habituation. Blood levels of 0.5 percent is lethal. Alcohol has a degenerative effect on vital organs and produces a loss of self control due to its action on the brain.

Alcoholism : This is a social problem. The term is used for all those who are addicted to the use of alcohol to such a degree that it interferes with their health, personal relation, social adjustment and efficiency. The habitual indulgence of alcohol produces chronic alcoholism. The early symptoms are chronic catarrh in stomach, throat and larynx accompanied by skin affections. Fatty degeneration occurs in the liver and the arterial walls throughout the body. Cirrhosis of the liver is common in alcoholics. It may lead to impairment of memory, self control and higher mental activity. Tremor and hallucination is not uncommon.

Treatment of Acute Alcoholic Intoxication

Treatment consists of evacuating the stomach by means of stomach tube. In case of respiratory depression inhalation of oxygen may be indicated. Amphetamine may be used in case of profound coma. Administration of molar sodium lactate to reduce the edema of the brain and sedatives like paraldehyde, 4-12 ml by rectum is also indicated.

Treatment of Chronic Alcoholism

This requires psychotherapy for the craving for drinking. Amphetamine has also been used to overcome the depression following withdrawal of alcohol. Drugs used for the treatment of alcoholism are :

1. Disulfiram (antabuse)
2. Citrated calcium carbimide (Temporil)

    1. **Disulfiram (antabuse) :** Disulfiram or tetraethyl thiuram disulphide is used in the treatment of alcoholism because of the disagreeable symptoms which it induces when ingested concomitantly with alcohol. This drug inhibits hepatic aldehyde oxidase and elevates blood

acetaldehyde levels, the bad symptoms elicited have been attributed to the accumulation of this degradation product. Disulfiram interferes with enzymes which oxidize acetaldehyde. Disulfiram is administered orally in an initial dose not exceeding 0.5 gm daily. The usual maintenance dose is abont 0.25 gm, ranging from 0.125 to 0.5 gm daily. Treatment is continued uninterruptedly until the patient is capable of controlling his drinking behaviour. Disulfiram is absorbed slowly from the intestinal tract. It must be taken 12 to 24 hours prior to a dose of alcohol. Disulfiram following the ingestion of alcohol manifests flushing, sweating, palpitation nausea and vomiting. Drowsiness follows with recovery after a period of sleep.

Toxic effect : Cardio-vascular collapse is the most important toxic effect.

Precautions : The drug should be used with other measures, leading to emotional and social rehabilitation of the alcoholics.

2. **Citrated Calcium carbimide :** This drug resembles disulfiram in its actions. It is lesss unpleasant than disulfiram. The reactions of the drug can be controlled by an antihistaminic.

4.12. STIMULANTS OF THE CENTRAL NERVOUS SYSTEM

Drugs that are used therapeutically to stimulate the CNS are known as analeptics. The use of analeptics depends on their capacity to stimulate the vital medullary centers when these are depressed. They act by antagonizing the action of depressants of these centers or by improving the metobolic ability of the brain.

Pentylenetetrazol ro Pentamethylene Tetrazol (Leptazol)

Leptazol acts primarily on the midbrain, medullary centers. It is effective in recovery from narcotic depression, especially that produced by barbiturates. In small doses it stimulates the respiration and the heart rate.

Nikethamide (coramine)

Nikethamide is a rspiratory stimulant acting through the carotid body. It also raises the blood pressure by stimulating the medullary centers. In large doses it produces excitement, tremors and convulsions. It is effective in respiratory depression of morphine and chloral. Nikethamide is used in a 25 percent aqueous solution. In emergencies it can be given intravenosly in doses of 1 to 5 ml as required. It is rapidly inactivated in blood system.

Caffeine

It is a purine derivative related to xanthine. The pharmacological actions of caffeine differ in the relative intensity of their action on various functions. Caffeine is the most potent central nervous stimulant of the group of xanthines viz Caffeine, Theoplylline and Theobromine. Theobromine exerts maximum effect on skeletal muscle and less on CNS. Theophylline is effective as a coronary dilator. Caffeine stimulates the CNS, in particular the part associated with physical function. It removes fatigue and drowsiness. It stimulates the higher nervous centers and manifests insomnia. Caffeine also stimulates respiration by its action on the medullary center. Caffeine is absorbed readily from the gastrointestinal tract and rapidly metabolized and excreted from the body after demethylation. A degree of tolerance is acquired on prolonged use of tea and coffee which are the main natural source for caffeine. Caffeine is used as citrated caffeine or as a donble salt cafteine with sodium benzoate. Both are soluble in water. Oral dose is 200 to 500 mg.

5

DRUGS FOR THE TREATMENT OF INFECTION AND CANCER CHEMOTHERAPY

Drugs used in the treatment of infections are the antimicrobial agents, sulphonamides, various antibiotics and the antiviral drugs. The selection of these drugs for therapeutic use depends on the susceptibility of the microorganisms to the drug. Microbial sensitivity and the drug's pharmacokinetic behaviour determines the choice of a particular antimicrobial agent for treatment of an infection. These agents are divided into various groups based on the mode of action of each agent used in the treatment of an infection, such as :

(i) Drugs that inhibit or activate enzymes that disrupt bacterial cell wall to cause the destruction of the pathogen are represented by antibiotics like penicillins, cephalosporines, cycloserine, vancomycin, bacitracin, miconazole and ketoconazole.

(ii) Agents which directly act on the cell membrane and on the cell wall sterols are represented by polyene antifungal agents like nystatin, amphotericin B.

(iii) Some drugs affect the function of bacterial ribosome to inhibit protein synthesis. The representative drugs are chloramphenicol, tetracycline, erythromycin and clindamycine.

(iv) Agents that can bind to the ribosomal substance to alter protein synthesis and kill the microbial cell are aminoglycosides like gentamicin, kanamycin, neomycin and streptomycin.

(v) Some drugs affect nucleic acid metabolism and can inhibit RNA polymerase which are DNA dependent, represented by rifampin, nalidixic acid and its derivatives and metronidazole.

(vi) Sulphonamides and trimethoprim block a particular step in the metabolism that are essential for the bacterial growth.

(vii) Antiviral drugs like vidarabine and acyclovir which are nucleic acid analogs can bind to the viral enzyme to produce antiviral action by blocking DNA synthesis.

5.1. PENICILLINS AND CEPHALOSPORINS

The penicillins for more than three decades have remained one of the most useful and versatile antibiotics. The term antibiotic has been derived from the phenomenon of antibiosis which refers to the ability of one microorganism to interfere with the growth of another microorganism due to production of specific diffusible metabolic products. These products are termed as antibiotics., The original most active antibiotic used in therapeutics was penicillin.

The penicillin derivatives exert their antibacterial activity by interfering with the synthesis of peptidoglycan by inactivation of transpeptidase enzyme that is essential for the final step of cell wall formation of growing bacteria.

Penicillins are derivatives of 6-aminopenicillanic acid which differ in their side chain structure. The cephalosporins differ from penicillins only in central chemical ring structure. Synthetic cephalosporins are made by substitution on both ends of the central ring structure. The important disadvantage of penicillins and cephalosporins is manifestation of bacterial resistance due to formation of bacterial enzyme called penicillinase and cephalosporinase which inactivate the drug by opening the beta lactam ring.

All penicillins are bactericidal. Hower, individual penicillins can be sensitive to either gram-positive or gram-negative bacteria or can have a broader spectrum of activity. The outstanding disadvantage of penicillins is the hypersensitivity reaction. The following are the penicillins commonly used in therapeutics.

Benzyl Penicillin (penicillin G)

This drug is inactivated by gastric acid so it is administered as injection, the peak blood concentration is obtained within 15 minute but 60 to 90% of the drug is eliminated within an hour. A combination with procaine viz. Procaine penicillin makes it a repository form with a duration of action which may last for about 12 to 24 hours.

Benzyl penicillin is the antitbiotic of choice for the treatment of pneumococcal, meningococcal and streptcoccal infections. It is very effective in syphilis and gonorrhoea. The dose of 300 mg, 6 hourly suffices for most infections which are sensitive to penicillin.

Phenoxymethyl Penicillin

Phenoxymethyl penicillin is orally active as this agent is gastric acid reistant. The drug can be administered as tablets or suspension in a dose of 500 mg 4 to 6 hourly. The drug is to be given before meals to assure maximum absorption. It is a drug of choice in upper respiratory tract infection and can be used prophylactically for a long time following an attack of rheumatic fever.

5.2. PENICILLINASE RESISTANT PENICILLINS

To overcome deactivation of penicillin by penicillinase the penicillinase resistant penicillins have been developed. This group of drugs include *Methicillin, Oxacillin, Cloxacillin,* and *Dicloxacillin.* These semisynthetic penicillins are used for infections arising out of penicillin resistant organisms. Oxacillin and cloxacillin have similar pharmacological and pharmacokinetic properties and can be given parenterally or orally. They are highly protein bound and more potent than methicillin. The usual dose is 500 mg 6 hourly but can be given upto 1gm every 4 hourly if the infection is virulent.

5.3. BROAD SPECTRUM PENICILLINS

Ampicillin

Ampicillin is one of the first broad spectrum penicillins. Ampicillin is relatively acid stable and is well absorbed from the gut, with a peak plasma level approximating 3 µg per ml two hours after the administration of 500mg. The serum half life is prolonged in uremic patients. Excretion of the drug is primarily via kidneys and high urinary concentration is attained after a dose of 1 to 2 gm per day in adults. The drug is also excreted in the bile. Both oral and parenteral preparations are available. The drug is used in urinary tract infection, bronchitis, bacterial dysentery and typhoid fever. Skin eruptions and diarrhea are the common side effects.

The other durgs belonging to this group are *Amoxicillin, Carbenicillin* and Clavulanate amoxycillin combination. Clavulanic acid is beta lactamase inhibitor with weak antibacterial activity.

Amoxycillin

Amoxycillin is analogous to ampicilin. It is an acid stable, well absorbed oral broad spectrum penicillin. It is rapidly and completly absorbed from the oral route and peak blood level is twice that of ampicillin at the same dosage. It is mainly exerted in urine. The adverse reactions are same as that of ampicillin with fewer gastrointestinal symptoms.

5.4. THE CEPHALOSPORINS

They closely resemble the penicillins differing only in the central ring structure. Synthetic cephalosporins are made by substitution at both ends of the ring structure. The machinism of action is the same as that of penicillins. The cephalosporins are generally excreted unchanged in the urine. They are acid resistant and resistant to penicillinase.

Cephalexin and Cepradine

Cephalexin and Cepradine are oral cephalosporins. Both drugs are absorbed well and after oral administration peak plasma levels at one hour after a single 500 mg dose are 18 ug per ml and 16 ug per ml. respectively. Both drugs are insignificantly bound to serum proteins. The serum half life is between 35 to 60 minutes. Suspension is better absorbed than capsules, absorption may be impaired with severe infections. They are effective from 250 to 1gm. every 6 hourly depending upon severity of infection and renal function.

Cefazolin sodium. cephradine and cephalexine are the cephalosporins that are mainly used in the treatmet of bone infections, septicemia, skin and soft tissue infections.

Adverse effects : Allergic reactions, diarrhoea, nausea and nephrotoxicity.

Drug interactions : Risk of renal damage if used in conjunction with aminoglycoside antibiotics. Frusemide can increase blood levels of some cephalosporins.

Cefoperazone

It is a semi-synthetic antibiotic, effective against a wide variety of organisms, and is resistant to degradation of beta-lactamases.

It is eliminated largely by the liver, so dosage adjustment is not required in renal failure as in the case of other cepholosporins. It is indicated in infections of respiratory tract, urinary tract, peritonitis, speticemia bone and joint infections, pelvic inflammatory disease and infection of the genital tract.

It produces its effect like other beta-lactum antibiotics by interference with bacterial cell wall synthesis.

Cefoperazone produces a high serum and urine level after a single dose of the drug which is between two to four grams per day to be given in equally divided doses every 12 hours. It can be used concomitantly with other antibiotics. However solutions of cefoperazone and aminoglycoside antibiotics show physical incompatibility and so should never be mixed while injecting. The mean serum half life of cefoperazone is about 2 hours dependent on the route of administration. It is excreted in the bile and urine.

The serum half life is prolonged in hepatic dysfunction and urinary excretion is affected.

The adult dose is 1 or 2 gram every 12 hours and in infants and children the dose is 50 to 200 mg/kg/day.

Adverse Reactions

The drug is contraindicated in patients known to have hypersensitivity to Cephalosporins and penicillins. The drug can decrease the hemoglobin concentration, can show transient eosinophilia and hypoprothrombinemia as hematological adverse reaction of the drug.

Altered bowel habits have also been reported as an adverse effect.

5.5. AMINOGLYCOSIDE ANTIBIOTICS

These are streptomycin, kanamycin, amicacin, gentamycin and neomycin which have similar common adverse effects and are not absorbed from oral route. So for systemic effect they are administered parenterally.

All aminoglycoside antibiotics act directly on the ribosome by interference with the attachment of messenger RNA and so there is abnormal protein synthesis thus producing bactericidal effect. The dose of streptomycin is 1gm a day.

Bacterial endocarditis, an inflammatory alteration of endocardium most commonly involving a heart valve dysfunction can be treated with streptomycin in combination with penicillin G. *Kanamycin is* active against gram negative organisms and resistance develops much slowly than streptomycin.

Gentamicin is the antibiotic of choice in septicaemia, burn induced skin and soft tissue infections and the infections of the central nervous system and the respiratory system. The dose being 3mg/kg body weight in a day in three equal divided doses which can be increased up to 5mg/kg/day in severe infections.

Concurrent use of gentamicin with diuretics and neuromuscular blocking drugs are to be avoided.

Neomycin : This is too toxic for systemic administration, however, application for topical use is indicated in skin and eye infections.

Adverse effects : All aminoglycoside antibiotics are ototoxic and nephrotoxic so adjustment of serum level by its blood level measurements can prevent toxicity and ensure therapeutic blood level.

Drug Interactions : Ototoxicity increases with ethacrynic acid and frusemide in renal failure and nephrotoxicity with methicillin.

5.6. TETRACYCLINES

The tetracyclines are polycyclic naphthacenecarboxamide derivatives which produce their effect by inhibiting protein synthesis by binding to ribosomes. They penetrate bacterial cell membrane readily due to active transport systems present in the microbes. Absorption of tetracyclines from the gastrointestinal tract is incomplete and is especially hindered by food, milk and antaacids like aluminium hydroxide and calcium and magnesium salts which form chelates with tetracyclines. Dose is 1g in 2 or 4 divided doses. *Doxycycline is* the only tetracycline that does not form chelates with calcium and food does not interefere with its absorption. However iron is incompatable with doxycyeline as it forms insoluble complex. Tetracyclines undergo enterohepatic circulation; excretion occurs via kidney and in feaces. Tetracyclines are effective in Gram-positive as well as in Gram-negative microbes causing infections. However Gram -positive bacteria produce bacterial resistance quickly. Tetracylines inhibit Entamoeba histolytica. The preparations of tetracycline are *chlortetracycline, oxytetracycline and demeclocycline* which differs from the other two in that it produces higher and prolonged therapeutic blood level. The safest tetracycline is doxycyclin with increased gastrointestinal absorption and 90% of it is excreted in feaces. So it can be safely administered for infections in patients with renal insuficiency. Tetracyclines are safe antibiotics with few side effects. The commonest is diarrhoea which stops if drug is discontinued. Tetracyclines chelate with calcium and are deposited in developing bone and teeth causing brown discoloration, so it is contraindicated in children and pregnant women.

Side effects : Gastric disturbances, photosensitivity, rash, retardation of bone growth and tooth discolouration, when given to pregnant women and children under 8 are the common side effects of tetracyclines.

Drug interactions : Absorption of tetracyclines is reduced by lron antacids and milk. Blood levels are affected by phenytoin, and carbamazepine. Lithium toxicity increases with tetracyclines.

5.7. CHOLARAMPHENICOL AND MISCELLANEOUS ANTIBIOTICS

This has a wide range of activity and is very effective in enteric fever. The daily dose is 1 to 3gm, and can be given orally since it is well absorbed from the gastrointestinal tract. It is well distributed in body fluids and can reach therapeutic level in cerebrospinal fluid. It is metabolized by liver and excreted in the urine.

Chloaramphenicol eye drops and ointments are used in purulent conjunctivitis.

Toxic effects are dose dependent blood dyscrasias and bone marrow depression which can cause aplastic anaemia. In new born it can give rise to grey baby syndrome, a state of acute circulatory failure due to inadequate metabolic conjugation of the drug.

Erythromycin is effective against gram positive organisms, and produces its effect by inhibiting protein biosynthesis. It is absorbed from the gastrointestinal tract and diffuses in all body fluids except CSF. Erythromycin estolate is resistant to gastric acid and is used in a dose of 250 to 500 mg 3 to 4 times a day. It is used in patients that are allergic to penicillin. Erythromycin has a very low incidence of side effect. It is useful in tonsillitis, bronchitis, whooping cough, and summer boil.

Drug interactios : Erythromycin can affect the metabolism of theophyllin group of drugs leading to its toxicity. Erythromycin also increases the effect of oral anticoagulants and digoxin.

Roxithromycin : It is a long acting macrolide belonging to erythromycin group. It is used in respiratory tract infection. Skin and soft tissue infections and genitourinany infections. The dose is 150 mg twice a day. Other effects are similar to erythromycin.

Vancomycin : This antibiotic is not absorbed so it is given intravenously. Vancomycin is a complex glycopeptide which gets distributed in all body fluids including the CSF. The antibiotic inhibits the bacterial cell wall synthesis and is bactericidal. It is effective against Gram-positive bacteial infections. This is effective against penicillin resistant organisms. The main toxic manifestations like ototoxicity, nephrotoxicity and hypersensitivity reactions limits its use in serious infections; the route of choice being intravenous therapy.

5.8. ANTIFUNGAL DRUGS

Fungal infections can be superficial involving skin and mucous membrane or systemic which are extremely difficult to cure. The main antifungal drugs are Amphoterecin, Griseofulvin, Ketoconazole, Miconazole and Nystatin.

Amphotericin is the most important antibiotic for the treatment of systemic fungal infections. This is a polyene antibiotic which binds to ergosterol present in membrance of the fungi and yeast and produces fungistatic and fungicidal action. Amphotericin lyophilized powder is available for intravenous infusion, the dose is gradually increased daily commencing with 1 mg. The drug is relatively less toxic and is the most important antibiotic for treatment of systemic fungal infections. It is a moderately toxic drug. The side effects are fever, vomiting, thrombophlebitis, and nephrotoxicity.

Griseofulvin gets selctively concentrated in keratin and is the drug of choice in the treatment of ringworms. It has an affinity for keratin and therefore, useful for treating mycotic infections of skin, hair, and nails. It is well absorbed from the gut and is given in a daily dose of 500 mg in adults. Skin infections respond quickly but nails require several months therapy. Griseofulvin binds to polymerised microtubules and is fungistatic. Griseofulvin is absorbed from oral administration and most of the drug is eliminated unchanged in feaces. It is to be given orally because it has little effect topically. Griseofulvin has relatively low toxicity. However urticaria, photosensitivity, gastrointestinal distress, hepatotoxicity and leukopenia are the possible adverse effects.

Nystatin is a polyene antibiotic which has fungicidal properties. The antiobiotic is poorly absorbed from the gastrointestinal tract. Its mode of action is similar to amphotericin. Nystatin is used as an oitment in the treatment of candida infections of the skin. Oral candidiasis (thrush) and vaginitis are treated by topical application.

Ketoconazole : This is a substituted imidazole fungicide which alters the membrane permeability by inhibiting the synthesis of ergosterol, the main cellular sterol constituent of fungi. Ketoconazole is well absorbed, orally 200mg a day is the dose in dermal mycoses, vaginal candidiasis and other systemic fungal infections. It is contraindicated in pregnancy and hypertension. The main toxic effects are hepatotxicity and hypersensitivity reactions. Ketoconazole has the potential to induce interaction with drugs which are metabolized by microsomal enzyme system.

Besides these systemic anti-fungal drugs there are a number of *topical anti fugal preparations*. The examples are :

Topical Preparations

(i) A 25% benzyl benzoate emulsión preparation used for scabies and pediculosis.

(ii) Clotrimazol 10mg per gram in a cream base can be used for all fungal infection of skin and nail.

(iii) Miconazole nitrate 2% w/w gel inhibits the growth of common dermatophytes and yeast.

(iv) Quiniodochlor 4 to 8% cream for all types of dermatitis.

(v) Gamabenzene hexachlor 1% lotion for scabies.

(vi) Topical steroid preparations like Beclomethasone 0.025% w/w cream; Betamethasone 0.12% cream for eczema.

5.9. ANTI-VIRAL AGENTS

These chemotherapeutic agents can kill the infective virus with out injuring the host cell. The most important development in making antiviral agents are :

(a) X-ray crystallography of the macromolecule of the virus and

(b) The study of dynamics of protein and nucleic acid with computational chemistry. The following antiviral drugs are in clinical use for specific virus families.

(i) **Idoxuridine :** Produces its effect by altered transcription following incorporation into the viral DNA. This causes altered protein production.

(ii) **Vidarabine :** Inihibits the viral DNA polymerase. Advantage of this agent is that it affects mammalian DNA to a lesser extent. It is effective in the treatment of herpes zoster in immunosupressed patients.

(iii) **Acyclovir :** This interferes with DNA chain termination following incorporation and inhibition of viral DNA polymerase. The drug is used for primary mucocutaneous herpes simplex and herpes genitalis infections.

(iv) **Amantadine :** It is a synthetic tricyclic amine that inhibits influenza-A virus by inhibiting the attachment and uncoding the virus. It is absorbed from the gut and excreted by the kidney unchanged. Dose related side effects are CNS disturbances and seizure, so it is not used in epileptics.

(v) **Azidothymidine :** This is 3' deoxy thymidine that inhibits the infective and cytopathic effect of human T-lymphotrophic and lymphadonopathy associated virus. It produces its effect by reverse transcription.

Anti HIV Agents

Anti HIV agents are meant for Chemotherapeutic intervention of AIDS. Availability of wide range of functional bioassay techniques for measuring antiviral activity has given rise to new chemical entities as potiential anti-AIDS agents.

So far drugs belonging to the neucleoside class of compounds are approved for the wide scale treatment of AIDS and AIDS-related problems. These agents are Nucleoside reverse transcriptase inhibitors, that is they have a common mechanism of inhibition of the important viral enzyme reverse transcriptase. Nucleoside inhibitors that are presently prescribed for the treatment of AIDS are :

(a) 3-azido 2'3'-dideoxythymidine (ATZ)

(b) 2'3' dideoxyinosine (DDI)

(c) 2'3' dideoxycytidine (DDC)

The mechanism of action of these drugs is linked to the process of reverse transcription that is central to the replication and pathogenesis of the viral infections in AIDS. So the inhibition of this key biochemical event in the viral life cycle provides the efficacy. All of them produce their inhibitory effect after undergoing in-vivo phosphorylation to generate a triphosphate derivative which result into activation of the drug. The nucleoside triphosphate complex thus formed compete for natural substrate and thereby inhibit reverse transcription.

Adverse effects : Drug related toxicity and emergence of viral resistance are, the drawbacks of these drugs. Toxic effects are macrocytic anemia, leukopenia and myopathy. In addition incidence of enemia, meningoencephalitis, ulceration and nail pigmentation have been reported.

5.10. SULPHONAMIDES

Sulphonamides have important therapeutic uses for number of infections specially in the treatment of urinary tract infections. The usefulness of sulphonamide has increased with the introduction of trimethoprim-sulphamethoxazole mixture which is a synergistic combination for bacterial infections. Currently used sulphonamides can be divided into the following groups based on its duration of action and uses.

1. Sulphonamides for systemic uses :

   (a) Short acting with half life of 4 to 8 hours. Short acting sulphoanamides are represented by *Sulphamethizole, Sulphasoxazole sulphachlorpyridazine* and *Sulphadiazine.* These are used for the urinary tract infection of E. coli, otitis media, etc.

   (b) Intermediate acting sulphonamides have a half life of 11 hours and

   (c) Sulphonamide which are long acting having a half life of more than 12 hours find very little clinical application.

2. Poorly absorbed sulphonamides such as *Phthalyl sulphathiazole* and *Succinyl sulphathiazole* are used only for intestinal infections.

3. Sulphonamides for topical use is *Silver sulphadiazine.* Sulphonamides get bound to the plasma proteins and only the free drug producs antibacterial effect.

   Sulphonamides compete with para amino benzoic acid for incorporation into folic acid which is essential for bacterial growth, that are susceptible to the drug.

Toxic Effects

Short acting sulphonamides have low toxicity, however as they are weak acids they show renal toxicity, the common complication is crystalurea giving rise to renal stones. Other effects are urticaria, blood dyscrasias, nausea vomiting. Alkalinization of urine by administration of bicarbonates increases the solubility of these drugs and can prevent the renal toxicity. The other toxic effects include hypersensitivity reaction commonly seen with long acting sulphonamides so they have lost clinical importance.

Trimethoprim Sulphamethoxazole Combination (Co-trimoxazole)

Mode of action of this combination is the inhibition of utilization of para amino benzoic acid by sulphonamide in the synthesis of folic acid while trimethoprim blocks the conversion of dihydrofolic acid to tetrahydrofolic acid by inhibition of the enzyme dihydrofolate reductase. So this preparation acts at consecutive steps in the inhibition of the bacterial metabolic growth.

It is effective against a large number of gram positive and gram negative organisms. It is used in the urinary tract infection, typhoid, para typhoid, upper respiratory tract infections. The usual dose is two tablets twice a day containing 80mg of trimethoprim and 400mg of sulphamethoxazole. Both the drugs are acetylated before exceretion and some is excreted unchanged in the urine.

Drug interaction : Trimethoprim may potentiate the effect of warfarin, prolong the half life of phenytoin and interfere with clearance of digoxin, proainamide, and tolubatimide. It can affect the renal function when given with cyclosporine.

Sulphonamides increase the blood level of phenytoin and tolubtamide. It may enhance hypoglycaemic effects of sulphonylurea. Adverse reactions of the combination are pruritus, skin rash, vomiting, and blood dyscrasias. It is contraindicated in pregnancy and renal insufficiency.

5.11. ANTI-TUBERCULAR DRUGS

The treatment of tuberculosis is to be done with an appropriate regimen suitable for individual patients. A combination of drug therapy is obligatory because single drug soon gives rise to resistant organism if used alone.

Primary chemotherapeutic agents for the treatment of tuberculosis are Rifampicin Isoniazid, Ethambutol, Pyrazinamide, Paraaminosalicylic acid (PAS), Thiacetazone and Streptomycin.

Selection of regimen is based on drug combination, e.g. isoniazid and rifampicin or refampicin and pyrazinamide. The combination acts by killing the rapidly growing bacilli. The treatment is long drawn involving more than one year.

The other drugs used are Ethionamide, Prothionamide, Amikacin and cycloserine. They are indicated against some atypical mycobacteria.

Rifampicin

The drug belongs to a group of complex macrocyclic antibiotics and is used in the dose of 450 to 600 mg. It inhibits the RNA synthesis in bacteria. It is well absorbed from the oral route and is distributed in all body tissues and is metabolized by the liver. To avoid drug resistance it is administered in combination with isoniazid or ethambutol. Untoward effects are very few. Coloring of the urine and sweat is commonly seen. Rifampicin induces liver microsomal enzymes and as a result it can reduce the effects of anticongulants and other drugs like tolbutamide, clofibrate, diazepam, and oral contraceptives. Blood level of refampicin is lowered by PAS, phenobarbitone and phenytoin, whereas probenecid increases the blood level.

The other side effects are durg rash, gastric upset. Occasionally liver dysfunction and jaundice can also be produced by rifampicin.

Ethambutol

Resistance to the drug occurs rapidly if not used in combination. Isoniazid 300mg with ethambutol 800mg combination tablets are used in pulmonary and extra pulmonary tuberculosis. It is well absorbed from the oral route and widely distributed in the body tissues including cerebrospinal fluid. The drug is excreted in the urine and feaces.

Toxic effect : Optic neuritis and visual disturbances which however, is reversible. Drug fever, drug rash, hypersensitivity reactions have been reported occasionlly. Ethambutol absorption is delayed or reduced by antacids like aluminium hydroxide.

Isoniazid

Isonicotinic acid hydrazide (INH) probably interfreres with cellular metabolism of an important constituent viz. mycolic acid of the micobacterial cell wall. The drug is well absorbed from the gastrointestinal tract and diffuses in all body tissues including the CSF. The plasma level is dependent on the rate of metabolism which is genetically controlled depending on whether the patient is a slow or fast acetylator. The drug is excreted in urine, slow acetylators have higher concentration of the unchanged drug in the urine. Adverse drug reactions are peripheral neuritis, nausea, vomiting, visual disturbances hepatitis, pyridoxine deficiency and hyperglycaemia. Drug interactions are seen as increased effect of phenytoin and PAS. It may cause hyperpyrexia, tremor with alcohol and hepatitis with refampicin.

Streptomycin

A combination of streptomycin I gm by intramuscular route plus INH 15 mg/kg body weight by mouth with pyridoxine 10mg twice a week is an effective inexpensive treatment to be given for one year. INH 300 mg and thiacetazone 150mg is also effective in absence of primary drug resistance. Sputum culture every six months is suggested to determine the occurence of drug resistance. Adverse drug reactions with streptomycin are ototoxicity, nephrotoxicity and hypersensitivity reactions which are the most common.

Pyrazinamide

This agent is effective in the treatment of tuberculous meningitis, because the concentration in the CSF is equal to that in plasma. It can prevent relapse. It is used in the dose 750mg. Adversee effects are arthralgia, hepatomegaly jaundiae.

Anti-leprotic Drugs

The agents that are used in the treatment of leprosy are Dapsone and Clofazimine. The other drugs that can be used is *rifampicin*.

Dapsone

This is the main drug used in the treatment of leprosy. Chemically it is a sulfone related to sulphonamide.

Dapsone is bacteriostatic. It produces its effect probably in the same way as the sulphonamides. The absorption of the drug is slow but complete from the gastrointestinal tract and the drug sustains a steady blood level because it undergoes intestinal reabsorption from the bile. It is excreted in the urine and requires minimum treatment for two years.

Untoward effects are methemoglobinemia, drug rash and anorexia.

Clofazimine

It is now used as a component drug in the multiple therapy of leprosy. It is a phenazine dye which probably inhibits the template function of DNA. It is absorbed from the oral route and accumulates in the tissues. Thus therapy is possible if individual doses are given in a gap separated by four weeks. Dapsone resistant human leprosy has shown good results with clofazimine in a dose of 100 to 300 mg, the interval between doses being determined from the individual response. The compound is also useful for chronic skin ulcer produced by mycobacterium. Unwanted effects are liver damage and renal dysfunction.

5.12. ANTHELMINTIC DRUGS

Drugs for threadworms

Mebendazole : It is a versatile anthelmintic effective against single or mixed infection . A small fraction of the oral dose is absorbed. Dose is 100mg single dose, 2nd dose is to be given after 2 weeks. Hook worm infection is treated with a dose of 100mg morning and evening for 3 days.

Side effects : No systemic toxicity has been reported. Sometimes abdominal pain and diarrhea may be seen if the worm manifestation is massive. *Contraindication* Not to be given to pregnant women.

Piperazine : The drug is effective predominantly on ascaris. It causes paralysis of the worm and expulsion is caused from peristalsis. A portion of the dose is absorbed and remainder is excreted in the urine.

Side effects : Occasional gastrointestinal upset. Neurologic effects and urticaria have been reported.

Contraindication : The drug is not to be given in epilepsy and renal dysfunction. It can cause neurotoxic effects.

Thiabendazole : It shows high degree of activity against nematodes. Dose 500mg to be given after meals. Maximum daily dose is 3g.

Side effects : Anorexia, vomiting, dizziness and epigastric distress. It can cause giddiness and abnormal sensation in eyes. Decrease in pulse rate and systolic blood pressure and lymphadenopathy has also been reported.

Contraindications : The drug is not to be used in hepatic dysfunction and in patients with CNS complications.

Ascaricides

Levamisol : The drug is extensively metabolized in liver. Urinary excretion of unchanged levamisol is very low. Dose 50 to 150 mg is sufficient to control ascaris infection. The drug has few side effects, however minor gastrointestinal disturbances and CNS effects like dizziness, insomnia and confusion have been reported.

Taenicides

Niclosamide : The drug is effective in the treatment of tapeworm infections. It causes disintegration of worm segments, it should be followed by a purge to identify colex. The recommended dose is 2g for adults and children over 8 years of age in two doses of 1 g each.

Drugs used in the treatment of Filariasis

Diethylcarbamazine : It is a piparazine derivative effective for filarial infection. The usual dose is 2mg/kg of the citrate salt three times a day for 7 to 21 days. It can produce severe allergic manifestations.

ANTIPROTOZOAL DRUGS

The protozoal infections are malaria, amebiasis, giardiasis, trichomonaisis and leishmaniasis. The drugs used against these infections are antiprotozoal agents which are specific for different individual infections.

The protozoal organisms of the genus Plasmodium viz. P. falciparum, P. vivax and P. malarea are the causative malarial parasites. The female anopheles mosquito is the vector. The life cycle of the malarial parasite can be divided into the following phases :

   I. Sporozoite phase-Sporozoites are inoculated by anopheles mosquito into the bitten individuals.

   II. Primary tissue phase-Parasite penetrates into red blood cell and then gets localized in the liver tissue. In this phase it is first found as tropozoit and then matures into schizont. In this process the parasitized red blood cells burst which is followed by chill and fever. The antimalarial drugs have no effect on sporozoits. They only produce their effect on schizonts, hence known as schizonticides.

5.13. DRUGS USED IN THE TEATMENT OF MALARIA

I. **Quinine** is an alkaloid obtained from cinchona. Adult dose is 650 mg T.D.S. for 10 days. Oral absorption is good but can also be given as intramuscular injection. The plasma protein binding is 90% and $t_{1/2}$ is 16 hours. It is a rapid schizonticide and is effective gametocytocidal in plasmodium vivax , ovale and malaria. It has no action on the liver stage development of the parasite.

Toxicity : The minor toxic manifestation is bitter taste, the others are cinchonism nausea, vomiting, hearing loss and postural hypotension. The major toxiceffects are cardiac arrhythmias, hapatitis and neuromuscular paralysis.

II. **Chloroquin :** Tablets are available in the strength of 250 mg as phosphate which is equal to 150 mg of the base. The usual dose is 1g (600mg of the base) followed by 0.5g for two days. Total dose is 2.5g.

   The dose for prophylaxis is 5mg of the base/kg/week upto 300mg maximum. It is sensitive to plasmodium falciparm, malaria, vivax and ovale. It can be resistant to plasmodium falciparum. The oral absorption of chloroquinm is good with a very long $t_{1/2}$ It is a rapid schizonticide, but has no action on liver stages of the parasitic development.

Toxicity : It produces bitter-taste, otherwise it is a well tolerated agent. It can produce nausea, dysphoria, postural hypotension, accommodation difficulties and skin rash. In acute toxicity it may show retinopathy and cardiac myopathy.

III. **Primaquin :** The usual dose is 15mg of the base. It is adminstered daily for 14 days. Oral absorption is complete and the plasma $t_{1/2}$ is about seven hours. Primaquin eradicates exoerythrocytic forms of plasmodium vivax and ovale very effectively. It is gametocytocidal against plasmodium falciparum. *Toxic effects* are nausea, vomiting, diarrhea, abdominal pain. The most serious side effects are hemolysis and methemoglobinemia. Massive hemoysis have been reported in subjects with severe glucose-6-phosphate dehydrogenase deficiency.

IV. **Pyrimethamine :** Tablets containing 25mg in combination with 500mg of sulphadoxine is administered as the usual dose every 12 hours for 3 days. Pyrimethamine is an inhibitor of diydrofolate reductase of malarial parasite. However resistance develops quickly, Only used for prophylaxis and treatment of plasmodium falciparum resistant to chloroquin. *Toxic effects* The drug is well tolerated, however there are reports of megaloblastic anemia, pancytopenia and pulmonary infiltration.

V. Mefloquin : Used for treatment and prophylaxis of multidrug resistant falciparum malaria. Dóse 25 mg/kg/day orally.

5.14. ANTIAMEBIC DRUGS

Amebiasis is an infection of large intestine produced by *Entamoeba histolytica*. It can be symptomatic intestinal amebiasis or hepatic amebiasis with liver involvements. Drug treatment is aimed to relieve symptoms. The effective amebicides are tabulated below :

Table 5.1

Drug	Dose	Side effects
Diiodohydroxy quinoline	650 mg t.d.s upto 3weeks	Nausea, abdominal cramp In rare case it can cause sub-acute myelo optic neuropathy (SMON)
Metronidazole Tablets; 200, 500 mg I.V. infusion 5 mg/ml	500 mg t.d.s. for 10 days	Nausea, metallic taste, head-ache, peripheral neuropathy. Contraindicated in CNS dis-ease. Dose is reduced in hepatic disease.
Tinidazole Tablets; 300; 500 mg It has a longer half-life than metronidazole.	500 mg t.d.s for 10 days	Toxic effects are mild vomit-ting, pruritis,
Diloxanide furoate (furamide/an/ester hydrolyzed to diloxanide)	500 mg t.d.s for 10 days	Toxic effects are mild. vomiting pruritis, urticaria reported occasionally.
Emetine (alkaloid Ipecac) used for amebic hepatitis and amebic abscesses.	1mg/kg/ day I.M. up to 60 mg upto 5 days	Toxic effects are on cardiac and skeletal muscles.
Secnidazole (half-life about 25hrs) used for intestinal amoebiosis, Giardiasis, Trichomonal vaginitis.	2 gm single dose	Vomiting, pruritis

5.15.   ANTICANCER AGENTS

A group of different agents have been found to be effective in cancer chemotherapy. The major class of antineoplastic agents that are available for therapeutic use arise out of alkylating agents, antimetabolites, plant alkaloids and hormonal agents. These agents are toxic to proiflerating cells. However, all anticancer drugs are almost equally toxic to normal proliferating cells, as well as to tumor cells. It is important to note that gastrointestinal epithelium and hair follicles are composed of highly proliferating cells, so all anticancer drugs produce their toxic effect on the hair follicles and gastrointestinal physiology in particular. The same is applicable for the hematopoietic organ, and the cells of immune system. So nausea vomiting, anemia, alopecia and immunosuppression are the most common side effects of all cancer chemotherapeutic drugs.

General Considerations for Cancer Chemotherapy : There are nearly hundred different types of cancer. Each have different response to a given anticancer drug. Effect of an agent depends on degree of tumor cell specficity, its location, size, and other biochemical factors. It has been found that individual cancer cells become soon insensitive to a specific drug, so a combination of anticancer agents with different mechanisms of action is used in therapeutic practice in an attempt to destroy all the malignant cells. Anticancer agents kill a constant fraction of tumor cells. So in an attempt to eliminate all the malignant cells cancer chemotherapy is required as an adjunct to surgery or radiotherapy.

It has been found that all normal and cancer cells grow through discrete phases and they may be represented as Mitosis or M-phase and DNA synthesis or S-phase. Besides these there is a resting phase and an interphase which is the period between the episodes of mitosis. Most antitumor agents can be phase specific or phase non specific. Phase specific agents act at a specific phase of the cell cycle, for example some can kill cells at only S-phase that is DNA synthesis phase. On the other hand phase non specific drugs kill proliferating cells but do not act on cells at a specific phase in the cell cycle.

Toxicity and dosage of anticancer drugs : Anticancer drugs have low therapeutic index with narrow margin of safety so the dose of the drug is not calculated on the convention of body weight as done for other drugs. It is calculated on the basis of patient's body surface area expressed in square meters. All anticancer agents are moderately selective to tumor cells hence they show the following common adverse effects;

(a) Bone marrow depression

(b) Gastrointestinal effect such as bleeding, ulcers, vomiting

(c) Alopecia

(d) Nephrotoxicity

(e) Immunosuppression.

Classification of anti cancer drugs : Different classes of agents that are used for the chemotherapy of cancer are :

(a) Alkylating agents

(b) Antimetabolites

(c) Natural products

(d) Miscellaneous agents.

Alkylating Agents

Mechlorethamine is a prototype nitrogen mustard alkylating agent and is phase nonspecific in its effect. It produces a reactive carbonium ion to induce DNA cross linking and mispairing of bases and depurination, to produce an effective DNA damage that can be subject to repair by enzymes. It is used in Hodgkin's disease in combination with other agents. It is given intravenously followed by rapid saline infusion as it may cause tissue damage if otherwise administered. Its half life is about 10 minutes and is proliferation independent.

Cyclophosphamide is a nitrogen mustard that can be given orally as well as parenterally. It is a potent immunosuppressant so it is used for control of rejection of transplanted organs.

The drug is activated in liver by mixed function oxidase system into phosphoramide mustard which produces cytotoxicity. The metabolites are excreted by the kidneys. The leukocyte count is the guiding factor in dose adjustment. Unlike other nitrogen mustards this drug rarely induces thrombocytopenia and finds its therapeutic use in a wide variety of neoplastic disorders. Major side effects are induction of pulmonary fibrosis and cardiomyopathy on prolonged use.

Chlorambucil is the slowest acting nitrogen mustard. It finds its use in malignant lymphomas. This drug is also well absorbed from the gastrointestinal tract and is completely metabolised. The side effects are similar to other nitrogen mustards.

Nitrosoureas : These agents in aqueous medium decompose to alkylating and carbamylating intermediates. The effects of nitrosoureas are due to alkylation of DNA and carbamylation of lysine residues on proteins. *Carmustine and lomustine* are the two nitrosoureas of which the former is used in tumors of brain and meningeal leukemia because of high lipid solubility allowing the agent to cross the blood brain barrier. *Lomustine* has been used to treat primary neoplastic disease of the brain, kidney, stomach, colon, and lung.

Alkyl sulphonates : This group is represented by the drug *Busulfan*. The drug has an alkyl-oxygen bond. The cleavage of this bond produces an electrophile which forms intrastrand DNA cross-links and stops the multiplication of cells. The drug is absorbed orally and eliminated in the urine as methanesulphonic acid.

Side effects are myelosuppression, endocrine dysfunction, rapid purine catabolism, and skin pigmentation.

Triazenes : *Dacarbazine* is the prototype of this group. It is N-demethylated by the liver to act as an alkylating agent. The methyl carbonium ion formed can methylate DNA, RNA and protein. It is most effective against malignant melanoma a tumor composed of melanin pigmented cell. Side effects are similar to other alkylating agents.

Antimetabolites

These drugs have structural similarity to natural substances such as nucleoside, aminoacids or vitamin. They compete with natural substrate for the active site on an essential enzyme or for the receptor; thus if incorporated into DNA or RNA it can disrupt cellular function.

Methotrexate is a folic acid analog which inhibits dihydrofolate reductase that catalyses the formation of tetrahydrofolate from dihydrofolate. Tetrahydrofolate is involved in the synthesis of purine, thymidylate, methionine and glycine. So cell death is caused by the blockade of the biosynthesis of thymidylate and purine required for DNA synthesis. Methoterxate also inhibits

RNA and protein synthesis. The blockade caused by methotrexate can be intercepted by leucovorin (folinic acid) and thus thymidine can be converted to the required tetrahydrofolate coenzyme or to a thymidylate even in the presence of methotrexate. This allows the forcible recovery of nonmalignant cells with reduction of toxic effects of the drug.

The drug is absorbed from the oral route and eliminated by the kidney with out much metabolism. About 50% is bound to plasma proteins. Salicylates and sulphonamides increase the drug's toxicity by inhibiting renal excretion and displacement from plasma protein bound state. It does not penetrate blood brain barrier. However it can be administered intrathecally for cerebral leukemia. Disadvantage of this drug is that tumor cells may become resistant to methotrexate. It is used in combination with other drugs to treat acute lymphoblastic leukemia. Prolonged treatment can cause hepatic dysfunction. Urine must be made alkaline to prevent its renal toxicity.

Purine analogs : The two drugs belonging to this group 6-Mercaptopurine and 6-Thioguanine are therapeutically used. *6-Mercaptopurine* is an analog of hypoxanthine. This is converted to 6-mercaptopurine ribose phosphate by the enzyme hypoxanthine-guanine phoshoribosyltransferase to inhibit purine biosynthesis. In addition to this action the 6-mercaptopurine ribose phosphate is capable of inhibiting adenylsuccinate synthetase and inosinate dehydrogenase that are involved in various steps of purine biosynthesis. The drug is useful in the treatment of lymphoblastic leukemia and chronic myelogenous leukemia. After administration of 6-mercaptopurine 50% of the drug is excreted in 24 hours as 6-thiouric acid. About 20% is plasma protein bound. The major side effect is myelosuppression with other effects similar to any other anticancer drug. Hyperuricemia and hyperuricosuria may be produced by 6 mercaptopurine. Allopurinol (antigout drug) an inhibitor of xanthine oxidase can block hyperuricemia and hyperuricosouria. However allopurinol reduces metabolic inactivation of the drug therefore the dose of 6 mercaptopurine must be reduced in patients receiving allopurinol. *6 Thioguanine* is the other purine analog which has similar mechanism of action as that of 6-mercaptopurine producing its effect by inhibition of purine biosynthesis. The drug is used in the treatment of acute myelogenous leukemia. It is less hepatotoxic than 6-mercaptopurine.

Pyrimidine analog : The prototype for this group is 5 *flurouracil* and *cytarabin*. 5 flurouracil is metabolically activated to a nucleotide 5 fluoro 2 deoxyuridine 5 monophosphate. This inhibits DNA synthesis, by blocking thymidylate synthetase. Normally thymidylate synthatese transfers a methylene group from reduced folic acid to deoxyuridylate monophosphate to form thymidylate, the essential material for DNA synthesis. The cytotoxicity may also be attributed to incorporation of 5 flurouridine triphosphate (also metabolically formed) into RNA. Thus 5 flurouracil is phase non specific, killing cancer cells not only in the S-phase but also through the cell cycle due to its action on RNA formation. The drug is used in combination with other agents for the treatment of breast cancer. It is also used in carcinoma of cervix and prostrate. The drug is administered intravenously and metabolized by liver. It is well distributed throughout the body including the CSF. The major side effects are myelosuppression together with common toxic effects as seen with other anticancer agents. Neurologic untoward effects may be seen in some patients.

Cytarabine : This drug is activated by pyrimidine nucleoside kinase to nucleotide triphosphate which inhibits DNA polymerase thus blocking DNA synthesis. Cytarabine is given intravenously to treat acute myelogenous leukemia in combination with 6 thioguanine. It has a very short plasma half life.

Natural products

A wide variety of plants and lower organisms have yielded a number of chemicals that are used as anticancer drugs. All of them have complex chemical structures.

1. **Actinomycin D** or **Dactinomycin** contains two cyclic polypeptides that are linked by a chromophore. It is a phase non specific agent that binds to DNA and inhibits DNA directed RNA synthesis. The drug is rapidly removed from the circulation but remains in the body for a long period. It does not cross the blood brain barrier. It is used In combination with other agents. It is immunosuppressive and is used in organ transplant such as kidney transplants besides cancer chemotherapy.

2. **Anthracyclines** are represented by *doxorubicin* and *daunorubicin*. They contain amino sugar and anthracycline ring structure. The drug molecule, gets inserted in DNA molecules so they inhibit protein synthesis. Pharmacokinitics of both are similar, they are rapidly taken up by all tissues except brain. They have long plasma half life, which is common to anthracyclines. Anthracyclines are metabolized and excreted as hydroxylated conjugates. They are effective against acute leukemia and malignant lymphoma. They are administered intravenously. The main side effect can be more because of the cumulative action of the drug. It can cause cardiac damage besides other toxic effects that are manifested in cancer chemotherapy.

3. **Bleomycin** is a mixture of glycopeptides. Different types of bleomycins differ in their terminal amino positions. They interact with DNA, one portion of the drug molecule generating free radical which cleaves DNA at purine-guanosine-cytosine-pyrimidin-sequence. It is used in combination with other drugs. The plasma half life is about one hour and more than 50% of the drug is excreted unchanged in the urine. It is administered intravenously, It is most useful in the carcinoma of the skin. Pulmonary toxicity is seen with other effects.

4. **Mitomycin** has aziridine ring system in its structure . This is reduced by nicotinamide adenine dinucleotide phosphate (NADPH) and then it alkylates DNA. Therefore, it acts as an alkylating agent. It is very short acting and metabolised by liver. It is used in the treatment of carcinoma of stomach and cervix besides others. Major side effects are myelosuppression, dermal and pulmonary toxicity.

5. **Vinca Alkaloids :** *Vincristine* and *Vinblastine* have been derived from the plant periwinkle. Both compounds have complex chemical structure with only difference of an aldehyde group in vincristine but their clinical uses and toxicity are quite different. Both agents act by blocking proliferating cells as they enter the metaphase. Both the drugs bind to tubulin so the assembly of spindle protein which occurs during mitosis is blocked. Both drugs are metabolized by liver and excreted in the bile. A small amount can cross the blood brain barrier. Both the drugs are bound to the body tissues. The therapeutic use of

vincristine is against acute lymphoblastic leukemia and lymphomas. It is also effective in breast and cervix cancer. The main difference in the two drugs lies in toxicity. *Vincristine* causes less myelosuppression than *vinblastine*.

Both the drugs are administered intravenously. Unwanted effect of vinblastine is leukopenia. Vincristine may show neurological manifestation which· is controlled by dose adjustments. Other toxic manifestations are similar to any other anticancer agent.

Miscellaneous Anticancer Drugs

These drugs are represented by I. *Cisplatin* II. *Hydroxyurea* III. *Procarbazine* IV. *Tamoxifin and* V. *Hormones and hormone antagonists.*

Cisplatin

This is an inorganic complex of diamminedichloroplatinum. The cis-isomer is only active. It binds to DNA causing cross linking. It also binds to nuclear and cytoplasmic proteins. It is a phase nonspecific agent. Pharmacokinitic studies show that 90% of the drug is protein bound and has a long half life of nearly two days. It crosses the blood brain barrier to a very small extent. It is administered as an intravenous drip with simultaneous administration of manitol as diuretic to overcome renal toxicity because the drug is known to cause dose dependent renal tubular dysfunction. Besides, cisplatin can cause anaphylaxis and hearing loss.

Hydroxyurea

This drug inhibits ribonucleotide reductase, an enzyme essential to form deoxyribonucleotide involved in DNA formation. The agent is phase specific and acts at the S-phase of the cell cycle. It is effective in the treatment of chronic and acute myelogenous leukemia. The drug is rapidly absorbed from the gastrointestinal tract and about 20% of the drug is metabolized by the liver and rest is excreted by the kidney. It is administered orally as well as intravenously, however in renal dysfunction it is not administered intravenously. The major side effect is reversible myelosuppression and cutaneous reaction. The reactions are common to other cancer chemotherapeutic agents.

Procarbazine

This is a hydrazine derivative which undergoes auto-oxidation and forms hydrogen peroxide which leads to DNA degradation. It also inhibits RNA synthesis. The major use of the drug is in Hodgkin's disease (Malignant Lymphoma) in combination with other agents. It is administered by mouth. The major side effects are leukopenia and thrombocytopenia. Procarbazine is a MAO inhibitor so it can cause hypertensive reactions when taken with food containing tyramine (eg. cheese) and sympathomimetic drugs and tricyclic antidepressents. Procarbazine is rapidly absorbed from the gastrointestinal tract and distributes itself in all body fluids including CSF but is rapidly metabolized and about 40% is excreted in the urine.

Tamoxifen

It is triphenylethylene derivative with antiestrogenic activity. It has been observed that estrogen is required for cell proliferation in breast cancer and estrogen receptors have been found in breast tumor. Tamoxifen competes with estrogen for the cytoplasmic receptors. Thus it blocks the growth-promoting effect of estrogen dependent tumors. Tamoxifen is absorbed when administered orally. It undergoes hepatic metabolism. The uncommon side effects of this cancer chemotherapeutic agent are hot flushes and mild fluid retention. The other side effects are the same as other anticancer drugs.

Androgen and Androgen Antagonists

The growth of many tissues is influenced by hormone and some tumors continue to posses receptors for them. Lymphoid tumors have receptors for glucocorticoids, estrogen and progesterone. Hormones bind to receptors in cytoplasmic cell and nucleus, which is associated with structural change in the receptors that interact with DNA in the nucleus leading to variation in protein synthesis. Hormonal therapy for cancer is dependent on receptors required for cell multiplication. So hormones and antagonists have found their use as antineoplastic drugs. Androgens that have been used for breast cancer are flumoxymesterone, dromostanolone and testosterone. Antiandrogens such as flutamide and cyproterone have been used in prostatic cancer. Prednisone has been used in combination with other drugs in treatment of leukemias.

5.16 IMMUNO SUPPRESSIVE AGENTS

These drugs are used for prohylaxis usally in autoimmune diseases along with corticosteroids. They are represented by Azathioprine, Murine Monoclonal Antibody (Muromonab - CD_3) and Cyclosporine.

Cyclosporine : It is an eleven aminoacid polypeptide extrated from the fungus *Tolypocladium inflatum gams.* The amino acids in the molecule are N-methylated which makes it non degradable in the gastrointertinal tract.

Cyclosporine has specific immunologic action in comparison to other drugs of this group. Immunosuppressive action is mediated through inhibition of T cell function and may have a direct inhibitory effect on nuclear proteins that are essential for T lymphocyte activation.

The usual oral dose is 10 to 15 mg/kg daily. It can also be administered in I.V. fluids, however the dose should be one third of the oral dose. Cyclosporine is used in autoimmune disease and in altered immune reactions. It is specific in suppressing T-cell mediated rejections that are encountered in organ transplant surgery.

Major Toxicity

It can cause renal failure and hepatotoxicity. It can produce increased susceptibility to infections. Plasma creatinine concentration require monitoring because it is usually elevated during cyclosporine therapy. There can be development of lymphomas as seen with other immuno suppressive agents.

6

AUTACOIDS AND NON-STEROIDAL ANTI-INFLAMMATORY DRUGS

Autacoids are locally acting hormone like substances that originate from different tissues to modulate local circulation and influence the various processes of inflammation. Autacoid antagonists are of therapeutic importance. The autacoids that are involved in the disorders of immune mediated injuries are histamine and serotonin, which are decarboxylated amino acids. The other group is of angiotensin and kinins which are polypeptides. The most important group of autacoids which, structurally, are eicosanoids are the prostaglandins, leukotriens and thromboxanes.

6.1. HISTAMINE

This is derived from dietary amino acid histidine which on decarboxylation by the enzyme histidine decarboxylase produces histamine. Metabolism of histamine occurs through methylation and oxidation by monoamine oxidase to methylimidazole-acetic acid. Histamine is stored in different concentrations in the lungs, skin and intestinal mucosa. The release of histamine occurs from any antigenic stimuli. Phsiologically, food and vegal stimulation releases histamine stored in the mucosal cells of the stomach which regulates gastric secretion. Histamine in the lung and skin can also be released in response to an allergen which may give rise to rhinitis, asthma and urticaria. Besides these allergic responses histamine may have a role in growth and tissue repair. Histamine has been found to be present in large amounts in the hypothalamus in the CNS where it is thought to play the role of a neurotransmitter.

Release and storage of histamine : Histamine is stored in the mast cell. Antigenic substances cause the relaease of histamine when they bind to immunoglobulin (IgE) molecule located on the mast cell membrane. The release from the storage site is believed to occur because of stereospecific receptor perturbation which is activated by high intracellular calcium ion concentration dependent phospholipids. This histamine release can be inhibited by high intracellular levels of cyclic adenosine monophosphate. On the basis of studies of agonists and antagonists histamine receptors have been divided into two types viz. H_1 receptor agonist which mediates broncho constriction and intestinal contraction of histamine. Pyrilamine and ethylenediamine derivative is the prototype antagonist. 4 mythel histamine is an agonist for H_2 receptor which mediates gastric secretion and cimetidine is the prototype antagonist. Pharmacological action of histamine is different in different species of aminals. In human being it manifests bronchoconstriction and gastro-intestinal spasm as a result of activation through H_1 receptors. Histamine causes increased capillary permeability which can cause local odema.

Triple response of histamine : When a very small amount of histamine is injected intradermally it results in a typical classical triple response characterised by reddening at the site due to local vasodilation, formation of a disk of odema (wheal) at the site due to increased capillary permeability and a halo arround the wheal which has a bright crimson red flare. These three effects that is reddening, edema and flare are called the triple response of histamine. The cardiovascular effects of histamine are fall in blood pressure due to capillary and arteriolar dilation. Thus many drugs can induce fall in blood pressure due to release of histamine which can be severe at times.

Histamine is the mediator of normal gastric secretion. This property is used diagonstically to distinguish between pernicious anemia and other forms of anemia. In pernicious anemia there is loss of gastric parietal cells so there is no secretion of hydrochloric acid in response to histamine. Histamine is one of the many autacoids that take part in hypersensitivity reactions.

In allergic reactions histamine is relased because the allergen reacts with IgE located on the mast cell to induce a chain of biochemical reactions.

6.2. ANTIHISTAMINICS

Antihistaminic drugs exert their action directly on those peripheral effector cells which respond to histamine and is regarded as competivive antagonist. Antihistamine drugs combine with the same receptors in the cells as histamine. This prevents histamine from exerting its effect. The prominent group of agents that are used therapeutically to alliviate the symptoms due to allergy are the derivatives of ethanolamine, phenothiazine, ethylenediamine, alkylamine and piperazine. All of these agents block peripheral histamine (H_1) receptors.

These agents can be administered orally and are completely absorbed to reach peak plasma concentration within I hour after administration. The other prominent pharmacological effects for some of these drugs are anticholinergic effects because these drugs have affinity for muscarinic receptors. Some of the antihistaminic agents may also have affinity for dopamine and serotonin receptors. A number of antihistamincs have been demonstrated to be effective in preventing motion sickness e.g. meclizine hydrochloride, cyclizine hydrochloride which are piperazine derivatives used in a dose of 50 and 25 mg respectively 3 times daily. The main side effect of most antihistaminics is drowsiness. This can be explained because histamine is a neurotransmitter that plays a part in the regulation of sleep and wakefulness. Thus H_1 receptor antagonist that enters the CNS will affect sleep. Antihistaminics like promethazine can induce day time sleep. New antihistaminics have been developed that do not cause drowsiness e.g. Astemazol, Terfenadine, Loratidine and Cetirizine.

Cetirizine influences the late phase allergic reactions which are characterised by infiltration of inflammatory mediators particularly the eosinophils. This action is not related to its H_1 receptor antagonist activity.

The following is a summary of antihistaminic drugs commonly used in allergic disorders :

Table 6.1

Name	Dose	Contraindications
Astemizole	10mg once a day	pregnancy and liver disorder
Azatadine	1mg twice a day	In MAO therapy, hypertension
Buclizine	25mg thrice a day	—
Cetirizine	10 to 20 mg a day	Renal impairment.
Chlorpheniramine	8mg twice a day	—
Cyproheptadine	2mg twice a day	Glaucoma, peptic ulcer
Diphenhydramine	25mg thrice a day	—
Dimethindene	1mg thrice a day	Epilepsy and urinary retention
Embramine	25mg twice a day	—
Luvistin	20mg thrice a day	—
Methdilazine	8mg twice a day	—
Mebhydrolin	75mg twice a day	Glaucoma
Promethazine	10 to 25mg a day	—
Terfenadine	60mg twice a day	Pregnancy and lactation

All these drugs have common side effects. In therapeutic dose lassitude is most frequently seen. In chidren it can show CNS stimulation, excitement, ataxia, hallucination and even convulsion.

Drug Interactions

Antihistamines enhance CNS depressant effects of alcohol, benzodiazepins, hypnotics, tranquillisers, and narcotic analgesics. Antihistamines have been frequently given intravenously via infusion with other drugs. There can be a number of physicochemical incompatibilities.

6.3. SEROTONIN AND SEROTONIN ANTAGONISTS

Serotonin is 5-hydroxy tryptamine derived from tryptophan and are found in the enterochromaffin cells of the gastrointestinal tract. It is also present in the CNS where it is thought to be involved in the regulation of sleep, temperature and mood. It is a precursor of melatonin, a hormone that may influence endocrine functions. Methysergide and Cyproheptadine are the serotonin antagonists that are clinically used.

Methysergide

This is a semi synthetic ergot alkaloid derivative with out any oxytocic activity. The agent is useful prophylactically for the treatment of migraine. Methysergide is a competitive antagonist of serotonin that inhibits its vasoconstrictor and pressor effects. For prevention of migraine attack the drug is used in a dose of 6-8mg a day, starting with 2mg daily, gradually increasing to full therapeutic dose. Adverse effects are insomnia, nervousness and gastrointestinal irritation. Long term use can show fibrotic changes in pleuro pulmonary and cardiac tissues.

Cyproheptadine

This is a phenothiazine derivative which blocks H_1 receptors along with weak anticholinergic and CNS depressant effects. It is a competitive antagonist that blocks the vascular effects of serotonin. The usual dose is 12 mg in divided doses.

Eicosanoids

The name eicosanoids has been derived from the greek work 'eikosi, i.e. 'twenty'. These are a group of bioactive substances generated from a component of membrane phospholipids which primarily include arrchidonic acid a 20 carbon fatty acid viz. eicosatetraenoic acid. Prostaglandins were so named because it was first identified in seminal fluid, leukotriene was first found in leukocytes which are conjugated trienes and thromboxanes are synthesized in thrombocytes and contain an oxane ring. In the plasma membrane cells there is a large family of membrane receptors which when activated in response to a stimuli generate diacylglycerol which is then hydrolysed by diacylglycerol lipase. One of the fatty acids in diacylglycerol molecule is arachidonate the precusor of prostaglandins (PGs) leukotriens (LTs) and thromboxanes (TXs).

6.4. PROSTAGLANDINS

Pharmacological effects of prostaglandins are platelet aggregation and vasoconstriction. They are primarily of five types A,B,C,E, and F, the degree of saturation of the side chain of each being designated by subscripts 1,2, and 3. Individual prostaglandin is abbreviated PGE_2, PGF_2 and so on. Several prostaglandins serve as mediators of the inflammatory response, some stimulate uterine contractility and other smooth muscles. The following are the preparations of prostaglandins available for therapeutic use :

Carboprost (15 methyl PGF_2 alfa) is used for medical termination of pregnancy between 13th and 20th weeks and also for the treatment of post partum haemorrhage. Carboprost is contraindicated in cardiac, pulmonary, renal and hepatic diseases.

Alprostadil (PGE_2) is available for use in infants with congenital heart defects. *Prostacyclin* (PGI_2) is being studied for its ability to inhibit platelet aggregation and for its vasodilating effect. It has been used as heparin substitute in hemodialysis and cardiopulmonary bypass surgery.

Eicosanoid Antagonists

Glucocorticoids primarily inhibit phospholipase in a number of tissues to block the synthesis of prostaglandins, leukotrienes and thromboxane which explains their anti-inflammatory effect. Leukotrienes have a role in hypersensitivity reactions, their suppression explains the efficacy of glucocorticoids in allergic disorders.

The other group of agents that are used as eicosanoid antagonists are known as nonsteroidal anti-inflammatory drugs (NSAIDS). They inhibit cyclooxygenase enzyme, however there is a varying cyclooxygenase inhibitory effect of NSAIDS in different tissues.

6.5. NONSTEROIDAL ANTI-INFLAMMATORY DRUGS

Certain agents can block the activity of the enzyme cyclooxygenase and therefore the production of prostaglandins to show anti-inflammatory action. Besides, they have analgesic properties with out interacting with opioid receptors and are non-addicting. Some of these drugs have antipyretic effect. They also possess antiplatelet activity of varying degree. These group of drugs are used in the treatment of musculoskeletal joint inflammation, ankylosing spondylitis, osteoarthritis and any other painful inflammatory condition.

Ibuprofen

It is a propionic acid derivative and has anti-inflammatory effect equivalent to aspirin but it is a more effective analgesic than aspirin or paracetamol. It is a potent inhibitor of cyclooxygenase and prolongs the bleeding time because of antiplatelet effect. Ibuprofen is used in a dose of 400 to 800 mg four times a day. 90 percent of the drug is serum protein bound and there is very little first pass hepatic metabolism. The drug is absorbed completely on oral administration.

Side effects : Gastric bleeding, peptic ulcer, nausea, epigastric pain, renal papillary necrosis and depression in elderly patients are common side effects of Ibuprofen.

Neproxen and Ketoprofen

Both the drugs have similar action like ibuprofen. The dose of the drug is 250mg twice a day to be adjusted according to patient's response and tolerance. It is contraindicated in pregnancy and lactation and in children side effects are similar to ibuprofen. The dose of *ketoprofen* is 50 to 100 mg twice a day depending on patient's weight and severity of symptoms.

Piroxicam

Piroxicam is an oxicam derivative with a long half life. It is used in a dose of 20mg once a day. Piroxicam gel can be used in acute musculoskeletal disorders and osteoarthritis of joints as topical application. Toxicity of piroxicam is similar to all other NSAIDS with hypersensitivity reactions like erythema, rash, pruritus. *Diclofenac* and *Fenclofenac* are phenylactetic acid derivatives used in a dose of 100mg in a slow release preparation. It may have penicillamine like effect as well as intiinflammatory action. It has lowest incidence of side effects.

Oxyphenbutazone and Phenylbutazone

These are pyrazolone derivatives. Its long term use is avoided due to its toxicity. Both the drugs can be used in a dose of 100mg three times a day. The adverse effects are gastric irritation, fluid retention, and bone marrow damage.

6.6. DRUGS USED IN GOUT

Gout is a condition in which plasma urate level rises due to an error in purine metabolism and urate deposition occurs at selected sites in joints. Acute inflammation follows because of the ingestion of urate by poly-morphonuclear leukocyte. The drug that inhibits this process is *Colchicine*.

Colchicine is administered in a dose not more than 10mg which is absorbed from the oral route and produces blockade of cell division. Toxicity encountered on chronic administration are aplastic anemia and agranulocytosis. Inflammation of gout can also be treated with Indomethacin. *Indomethacin is a methylated indole derivative effective for control of pain and stiffness.*

Unwanted reactions are peptic ulceration, CNS complcations and heametological effects like blood dyscrasia, neutropenia and thrombocytopenia. The usual dose is 25mg three times a day. The other drugs used in gout are *Allopurinol, Probenecid* and *Sulphinpyrazone*.

Allopurinol

Allopurinol prevents the terminal step of uric acid synthesis. It is competitive inhibitor of the enzyme xanthine oxidase. Average daily dose is 100 to 200 mg and the dose is adjusted by monitoring serum or urinary urate. Allopurinol is 80% absorbed after oral dose. Allopurinol is effective in a low dose in lessening recurrent attack of gout. *Drug interactions of allopurinol is* seen as potentiating effect of oral anticoagulants and hypoglycemic effects of oral antidiabetics if concomitantly administered. *Adverse drug* reaction are rash, gastrointestinal disorder, fever, and renal failure. Peripheral neuritis and bone marrow depression may also occur.

Probenecid

This drug inhibits tubular reabsorption of uric acid at therapeutic dose of 1gm a day. It increases the uric acid excretion and produces a fall in serum urate. It has no analgesic activity. A metabolite of probenecid is also uricosuric.

Drug Interactions

Aspirin blocks the action of probenecid. So they are not to be given together. Adverse reactions are gastric disturbances and hypersensitivity reactions.

Sulfinpyrazon

Sulfinpyrazon and its hydroxy metabolite inhibits tubular reabsorption of uric acid. It also inhibits prostaglandin synthesis and interferes with platelet function. The drug is administered orally with meals. It is absorbed from the gut and excreted in the urine unchanged.

Drug Interaction

The therapeutic effects are reduced by salicylates and diuretics and enhances the effect of oral anticoagulants. Adverse actions are gastric discomfort and blood dyscrasias.

6.7. OTHER ANALGESICS AND ANTIPYRETICS

Salicylate group of drugs produce analgesic effect and also have antipyretic action. Peripheral vasodilation and abundant perspiration induce a prompt fall in body temperature in pyrexia. The representative drugs are *Aspirin, acetanilide, paracetamol,* and *phenazone.*

Salicylates

The most commonly used salicylate is Aspirin which eliminate the sensation of pain by altering the physiological reactions to pain through both peripheral and central mechanism.

It inhibits the synthesis of prostaglandin in the inflamed tissue to prevent sensitization of pain receptors to both mechanical and chemical stimuli. Other pharmacological effects are dose dependent such as higher doses of aspirin results in medulary stimulation producing hyperventilation. The other important effect of aspirin is gastric ulceration and haemorrhage because of increase in gastric secretion due to suppression of prostacyclin, the endogenous inhibitor of acid secretion in the stomach. Aspirin induces prolongation of bleeding time so it is recommended for prophylaxis of thromboembolism in a small dose of 300mg a day. It is recommended in myocardial infraction because of its antiplatelet activity as it can acetylate and inactivate cycloxygenase enzyme system which controls platlet aggregation. The renal effect of aspirin is dose dependent, at higher doses it promotes excretion of sodium urate but at low dose it decreases the same. So aspirin is not given with uricosuric drugs in the therapy of gout. The therapeutic use of aspirin is in relief of fever and headache. It is a drug of choice in rheumatiod arthritis due to its anti inflammatory and analgesic actions. It also provides relief in acute rheumatic fever. Aspirin is deacetylated after absorption into equivalent free salicylate. Absorption occurs from the stomach but the majority of the drug is absorbed from the small intestine.

Metabolic effect of aspirin are hyperglycemia and glycosuria when given in large doses. Large doses of aspirin stimulate steroid secretion by adrenal cortex. Aspirin binds to the serum protein to a lesser extent. An overdose of salicylates can be treated by making the urine alkaline. There is an increase in excretion of salicylates because of increased ionization which decreases the reabsorption of the drug at the renal tubules. However in case of salicylate poisoning along with other measures gastric lavage and dialysis is also required.

Available dosage forms of aspirin are tablets of different strength, buffered or enteric coated, and soluble aspirin which is better tolerated.

Paracetamol (Acetaminophen)

Paracetamol is the active metablolite of phenacetin. This is an effective analgesic antipyretic drug without anti inflammatory action. Paracetamol exerts no effect on blood pressure, respiration, gastric acid secretion or platelet aggregation.

Paracetamol is completely absorbed from the oral route. 3% of the drug is excreted unchanged and the rest of it is conjugated in the liver and is excreted in the urine. Paracetamol is available as tablets and as elixir in syrup base for use in children. Adverse effects are skin rash, renal tubular necrosis and kidney failure. In an over dose of the drug it can result in liver toxicity for which N-acetyl para benzoquinone a metabolite of the drug is thought to be responsible. Symptoms of nausea and vopmiting occurs with in 24 hours of toxic ingestion.

Ketorolac Tromethamine

Ketorolac is a cyclic propionic acid derivative available as the tromethamine salt. The tromethamine moiety enhances the aqueous solubility of ketorolac. The drug is used for the management of pain. Recommended usual initial IM dose is 30mg. Subsequent dosing should be 10 to 30mg every 4-6 hours as needed to control pain. Intramuscular ketorolac generally produces analgesia comparable to that of IM dose of opiate analgesic. However, unlike opiate analgesic ketorolac does not produce respiratory depression or physical dependence. Oral doses of 10mg of drug upto four times daily have been used for the management of moderate to severe pain. Ketorolac tromethamine is rapidly and completely absorbed following IM injection. The plasma half life is 5.3 hours in young adults and more in elderly subjects. More than 99% of ketorolac in plasma is protein bound over a wide concentration range. The primary route of excretion of the drug is in the urine. The metabolite para hydroxy derivative and the conjugate is also excreted through the same route.

The mechanism of action for the drug is atributed to its inhibition of prostaglandin synthesis. Adverse reactions are nausea, dyspepsia and gastrointestinal pain, dizziness, headaches, sweating and edema, liver function abnormalities,peptic ulcer and rectal bleeding. The drug is contraindicated in patients with active peptic ulcer and in aspirin sensitive persons. It is to be used with caution in hypertension, fluid retention and in kidney impairment. Ketorolac is distributed in milk so it should not be used in nursing mother.

7

DRUGS ACTING ON THE
DIGESTIVE SYSTEM

The digestive system comprises of the secretory organs like liver and pancreas and a muscular passage which is known as the gastrointestinal tract. Each portion of this tract has selective functions. Digestion of food is carried out by a number of enzymes secreted by different parts of this tract. The enzymes are mixed with food to be digested and after absorbtion the mixture is propelled out by a series of segmental and peristaltic movements.

Digestive system can have various disorders, therefore different kinds of agents are used in the treatment of digestive ailments.

7.1. DRUGS MODIFYING SECRETORY FUNCTIONS

Sialogogues : These are bitters that increase salivary secretion such as an infusion of quassia is used in a dose of 15 to 30 ml. The other drug is tincture of orange made out of fresh bitter orange peel used in a dose of 2 to 4 ml. *Stomacics, carminatives* and digestives are the agents that increase the gastric secretion and improve the digestion. The representative drugs are *quassia, chirata, orange and lemon peel* used as infusions or syrups or tinctures. *Digestants* are enzyme preparations containing *pepsin, pancreatin,* and *diastase*. These drugs are indicated in indigestion, dyspepsia, loss of appetite. Dehydrocholic acid obtained by oxidation of cholic acid and polysorbate 80 are used in *biliary stasis* and *steatorrhoea* respectively.

CONSTIPATION

One can find considerable variation in bowel habits in different individuals. Bowel movements are related to fibre intake and the function of colon which mixes and propels its content after the absorption of water and electrolytes. Colonic and rectal motilities are regulated by parasympathetic, sympathetic and enteric nervous system so any functional change in these nerve path ways will affect stool frequency. The motility of colon is dependent on bulk forming contents in the food. Presence of a particular amont of faeces in the rectum causes distension and leads to reflex contraction of the rectal smooth muscles and relaxation of internal anal sphincter. By contracting the diaphragm and abdominal muscle and relaxing external anal sphincter the stool can then be expelled, so defecation is a voluntary as well as involuntary process. There are number of causes of constipation such as :

   (i) Anorectal disorders like anal fissure, haemorrhoids.

   (ii) Colonic disorders like irritable bewel syndrome, tumours, iodiopathic slow transit constipation.

   (iii) Various neuromuscular causes like autonomic neuropathy, Parkinson's disease.

   (iv) Psychiatric diorders such as depression, anorexia nervosa.

   (v) Metabolic endocrine disorders such as phaeochromocytoma, hypokalemia and debility.

   (vi) Drug induced constipation can arise out of anticholinergic, antihypertensive drugs, iron, psychotherapeutic agents and others.

7.2. DRUGS USED FOR CONSTIPATION

Following Table 7.1 (at page 121) provides a list of selected group of laxatives and fecal modifiers used in treatment of constipation.

Senna Anthracene Purgatives

Two isomeric glycosides designated as sennosides A and B are

Table 7.1 : Drugs used as laxatives and fecal modifiers

Class	Drug	Doses	Main use	Side effects
Irritant stimulant	Senna anthracene glycoside.	Total senoside 5mg.	acute & chronic constipation	griping pain
	Castor oil	15 to 30ml	Strong laxative, produces fluid stool, evacuates bowel of gas for X-ray exams.	potential obstruction of bowel
	Phenolphthalin	60mg	As cathartic	Dermatitis
	Bisacodyl (Dulcolax)	5mg 10mg rectal suppositories	Empty lower bowel for endoscopic procedures; preparation for X-ray exams.	Rectal irritation from prolonged use of suppositories.
Bulk forming agents	Psyllium hydro-philic mucilloid (Isabgol)	7gm. in water.	Mild laxative	Obstruction of bowel
Saline cathartic	Magnesium sulphate Mixture of magnesium hydroxide (Milk of magnesia). Sodium phosphate, biphosphate (Fleet enema)	2 to 16 gm. 15 to30ml. 120ml rectaslly reflex, produces	Act locally by Changing osmotic pressure with in the gut, so increase peristaltic effect in short time.	Hypermagnesemia in renal failure
Wetting agents	Dioctyl sodium sulphosuccinate	50mg in syrup base	lessens strain of defecation	Not to be given with mineral oil
Lubricants	Liquid paraffin	15 to 30ml	Useful in infarction to avoid strainig at defecation	Reduces absorption of fat-so luble vitamins

the purified forms that are used to avoid the disadvantage of wide variation in potency of senna leaves.

The anthracene purgatives produce their effect only when they reach the large intestine. The interval between their administration and the evacuation of the bowel therefore, tends to be longer than most other purgatives.

Castor Oil

Castor oil while passing through the intestine is saponified by the pancreatic juice and the ricinoleates thus formed are irritant and cause purgation. Castor oil is absorbed from the small intestine and does not act on the large intestine directly. It can be administered in doses of 4 to 16ml in gelatin capsules or in emulsion form.

Phenolphthalein and its Synthetic Analogue Bisacodyl

Phenolphthalin and Bisacodyl are related chemically and have similar action. Phenolphthaline is insoluble in water. In the bowel it is dissolved by the bile and alkali and develops a mild irritant action in the small intestine and moves into the large intestine. Phenolphthaline is reabsorbed in the blood from the intestine and again carried to the liver and returned to the gut, so it can act for long time as a mild irritant as it is gradually eliminated in the the urine and stool and the action passes off.

Bulk Forming Agents

Agar a colloidal carbohydrate is indigestible, retaining water and acts as a demulcent and lubricant. It is useful in chronic constipation. It is administered as suspension in water in a dose of 4 gm.

Psyllium or Plantogo Seeds

It is available as powder from the Plantago ovata seeds. The seeds contain a mucilage which is indigestible. It swells in the gut and is used as a mild laxative. It is administered with water or fruit juice. It is used in a dose 4 to 7 grams.

Lubricants

Liquid paraffin is a hydrocarbon obtained from petroleum. It acts mechanically partly by increasing the bulk of the intestinal contents and partly by softening the contents and acting as a lubricant. It is used in a dose of 15 to 30ml in an emulsion form. It can retard digestion and interfere with fat soluble vitamin absorption.

Saline Purgatives

The saline cathartics used in therapeutics are sodium sulphate (Glauber's salt), magnesium sulphate (Epsom salt), double tartrate of sodium and potassium (Rochelle salt). The saline purgatives differ from the vegetable purgatives like senna or castor oil in not inducing irritation of the intestine. The main effect is retarded absorption. The contents of the intestine and the stool thus contain more fluid than usual and these salts are known as the saline cathartics. The catharctic action of magnesium sulphate is most powerful. The contents of the large intestine are more fluid than usual, and are passed down more easily towards the rectum. At the same time the weight and distention of the bowel induces increased paristalsis and the evacuation occurs. This increased peristalsis is due to the large amount of fluid contents, which arouses the peristaltic reflex. The first stool is of normal consistency but this is followed by profuse watery stool. The sulphates and tartrates are more frequently used. A single large dose is prescribed. Seidlitz powder is more agreeable to the taste. Sodium phosphate is prescribed for children as podwer to be given in jelly or milk. This can also be given in debility.

Wetting Agents

Dioctyl sodium sulphosuccinate by its surface active detergent action promotes the formation of oil-water emulsions which effects the stool. It is used as laxative in the form of capsules or as a syrup. The dose is 50 to 100 mg for an adult.

7.3. ANTIDIARRHEAL DRUGS

(a) Removal of bacterial toxins by adsorbents can be the basis for treatment of diarrhea. The common adsorbents are *kaolin and pectin*. They are used as a suspension in a mixture containing 20 gm of kaolin with 500 gm of pectin per 100ml of the suspension. The mixture is a very good adsorbent of the bacterial toxins; from the stomach and intestine which is a physical phenomenon. The colloidal mixture of kaolin and pectin provide the surface area for this process of adsorption.

(b) *Loperamide* produces antidiarrheal effect by reducing the motility of the intestine. Initial dose is 2mg followed by 2 mg after each loose stool up to 8mg in a day. The child dose is 0.1mg per kg. It is contraindicated in children below 2 years.

(c) Oral fluids

7.4. GASTRIC ANTACIDS

Simple hyperacidity can be counter-acted with a group of agents known as antacids. They act as palliative, protective and demulcents besides reducing hydrochloric acid secretion. Secretion of the gastric acid from the oxyntic cells of the stomach occurs in three phases.

(a) Basal secretion phase is interdigestive period during which acid is slowly and continually secreted at about a rate of 2.4meq/hour. This phase can be completely blocked by anticholinergic drugs.

(b) **Neurogenic phase :** The nervous stimulation is mediated by sight, smell of food and also by emotions like anger. Stimulation of vagus occurs which gives rise to highly acidic pepsin rich gastric juice. This phase is partially controlled by anticholinergics.

(c) **Hormonal phase :** In this phase gastrin is involved. Food or gastric distension stimulates oxyntic cells of stomach to secrete gastric hydrochloric acid. For various reasons the secretion of gastric hydrochloric acid can increase. Gastric antacids are the agents that reduce hyperacidity with out causing systemic alkalosis or rebound acidity. They cause less interference with digestive process, do not produce constipation or diarrhoea and are efficient in neutralising acidity for a long period. All these properties are met with non systemic, non absorbable, locally acting drugs like buffered aluminium hydroxide gel and magnesium trisilicate.

Aluminium Hydroxide

Dried aluminium hydroxide gel tablets or suspension in a dose of 600 to 800 mg is used for hyperacidity. The tablets are to be chewed before swallowing. Aluminium hydroxide combines with hydrochloric acid of the stomach to form aluminium chloride. In the intestine aluminium chloride is reconverted to hydroxide which effectively neutralises gastric acidity, inhibits peptic activity and reduces gastric secretion. Other aluminum salts that can be used for the same purpose are aluminium phosphate gel and aluminium glycinate.

Drug Interactions

Aluminium hydroxide reduces absorption of many drugs e.g. oral iron preparations, chlorpromazine, digoxin and tetracyclines. Adverse reactions are constipation and it binds to phosphates and reduces its absorption.

Magnesium Trisilicate

The hydrated silicon dioxide formed from the reaction of magnesium trisilicate and gastric hydrochloric acid is colloidal in nature and forms protective adherent coating over the stomach wall. The agent is long acting and requires a dose of 300 mg to 2gram a day to produce its effect.

Drug Interaction

Reduces the absorption of many drugs e.g. tetracyclines. Adverse reactions of magnesium ions can precipitate in presence of renal insufficiency.

Systemic Antacids

Besides these non systemic antacids there are systemic absorbable antacids such as *sodium bicarbonate and citrates*. These agents are immediately effective but are of limited use.

Solutions of *bicarbonate* are used as *systemic alkaliniser* in many conditions such as fever, gout, renal complications like cystitis, renal calculus etc. It can also be used for reduction of renal toxicity in sulphonamide and salicylate therapy.

Drugs used in healing of peptic ulcer

Treatment of peptic ulcer is based on the physiologic and pathologic role of histamine as a mediator of gastric secretion. It is known that histamine stimulates gastric acid secretion that cannot be blocked by standard antihistamines. However another group of agents which block the acid secretion of the stomach are the histamine H_2 receptor antagonists and forms the basis of treatment of choice for duodenal and gastric ulcers. The H_2 receptors are situated on or near the parietal cells in the stomach which mediate in the acid secretion.

Under normal condition the secreted acid of the stomach does not eat up the gastric mucosa because of mucosal resistance. This resistance is provided by surface epithelial cells. Normal turnover of the epithelial cell and the gastric mucosa provides the mucosal barrier that prevents gastric ulcers. Mucosal resistance can be reduced to give rise to gastric ulcers in many ways. These are :

(a) Prostaglandin inhibitors like aspirin group of drugs.

(b) Stress conditions which produce hyperacidity.

(c) Mucosal ischaemia in shock and other conditions.

Drugs which promote healing of peptic ulcers are H_2 blockers like cimetidine, ranitidine, famotidine, omeperazole. Sucralfate, carbenoxolone, dimethylpolysiloxane, and bismuth chelate, produce their effect in a different manner.

7.5. H_2 HISTAMINE RECEPTOR ANTAGONIST

The representative drugs *Cimetidine, Ranitidine and omeprazole*, all have higher healing rate and are well tolerated. With the discovery of 4-methyl histamine, an effective H_2 agonist, a number of compounds were synthesized that blocked the histamine induced acid secretion. These H_2 antagonists have the imidazole ring of histamine structure intact, modified only in the side chain which is longer. Addition of a sulphur group, gives rise to the drug Cimetidine. These drugs competitively block the action of both exogenous and endogenous histamine on gastric acid secretion in man.

Cimetidine in a dose of 200mg three times a day when given for 4 weeks heal duodenal and gastric ulcers.

Adverse effects of cimetidine is gynecomastia, oligospermia, elevated transaminase and mental confusion in aged. Nephiritis, hepatitis and pancreatitis have also been reported.

Drug Interactions

May potentiate the actions of anticoagulants, phenytoin,

theophyllin benzodiazepines, beta blockers and lignocaine.

Ranitidine in a dose of 150mg twice a day heals ulcers more quickly. It is more potent and much less toxic than cimetidine. The drug is absorbed from the oral route and rapidly excreted by the kidney. The dose has to be adjusted in renal insufficiency.

Drug Interactions

Antacids can hinder its absorption. The side effects are headache, dizziness, thrombocytopenia and hypersensitivity. The other group of drugs used in peptic ulcer are mucosal barrier strengtheners :

Sucralfate : It is effective in dose of 1 gm before each meal and bed time. It is sulphated sucrose with aluminum hydroxide. It acts locally by adhering to the ulcer and shields the mucosa from the acid and pepsin.

Liquorice derivative carbenoxolone : The dose is 50mg t.d.s. after meals. Side effects are salt and water retention, hypokalemia and rise in blood pressure.

Roxatidine

The chemical structure of Roxatidine is different from other H_2 receptor antagonist. Roxatidine acetate is converted into active metabolite in the small intestine and liver. Roxatidine inhibits the basal acid secretion as well as pentagastrin induced effect. In experimental animal models roxatidine is reported to have mucosal protective effects. It does not interfere with hepatic mixed finction oxidase system and has no effect on hepatic metabolism of other drugs. Roxatidine is well absorbed after oral administration and appears in blood within 45 minutes of its administration. Roxatidine is bound to the plasma proteins to an extent of 6 to 7 percent and the half life is about 6 hours. 90 percent of the drug is excreted in 24 hours.

The usual does is 75 mg twice daily, however dose reduction is required in renal dysfunction.

Adverse reactions of the drug are gastrointestinal disturbances, reduction in number of leucocytes, sleep disturbances. Roxatidine is contraindicated in pregnant and nursing women.

Omeprazole

This drug belongs to a new class of antiulcer agents with a different mode of action from that of other H_2 receptor blockers. It is a substituted benzimidazole derivative, with a specific inhibitory effect on the enzyme system that is regarded as acid pump present on the secretory surface of the parietal cells. Omeprazole blocks both basal and pentagastrin induced effects of acid secretion. The usual recommended dose is 20mg once daily in gastric and duodenal ulcers and other peptic disorders.

Drug Interactions

Omeprazole can prolong the elemination half life of diazepam, warfarin and phenytoin and so requires dose adjustment with concomitant administration. Adverse effects are nausea, diarrhoea, flatulence and skin rash. The drug is not administered in children and pregnant and lactating women.

8

ERYTHROPOETIC DRUGS AND DRUGS AFFECTING BLOOD COAGULATION AND BLOOD CHOLESTEROL

8.1. ANEMIA AND ITS TREATMENT

Anemia is the clinical state which is characterised by hematologic alteration from normal with a decreased heamoglobin in blood and corresponding reduction in the oxygen carrying capacity. The normal haemoglobin values in man is 14-18 gram percent and in women is 11.5-16.5 gm percent. To assess anemia heamoglobin, red blood cell count, percent volume of the packed red cells are measured. Anemia can result from various reasons, such as decreased red cell production due to deficiency of components like iron and coenzymes as in cyanocobalamine (vitamin B_{12}) and folic acid deficiency.

Anemia can be due to blood loss or malnutration. It is characterised as hypochromic microcytic anemia denoting iron deficiency. In this case iron availability decreases which is the major constituent of hemoglobin molecule. Some times porphyrin and globin availability may also decrease.

The other form of anemia is macrocytic anemia which is associated with the megaloblastic red cells in the bone marrow because of the deficiency of either vitamin B_{12} or folic acid. This deficiency produces an impairement of replication of DNA so nuclear maturation of RBC lag behind, with a result large red cells are produced in the bone marrow. Oral iron preparations such as ferrous sulphate, ferrous fumarate and ferrous gluconate are used in the therapy of iron deficiency anemia. The physiological role of iron contained in hemoglobin and other tissues like myoglobin, cytochrome catalase and peroxide are numerous. The most important role of iron is in the transport of oxygen by hemoglobin to the various tissues.

Absorption of Iron : Hydrochloric acid of the stomach converts ferric salts of food in the diet into free ferric ions which is then reduced by ascorbic acid into ferrous form. This is necessary because ferric form can not be absorbed. This is why most of the oral iron preparations used in iron deficiency are inorganic or organic ferrous salts.

8.1.1 Iron Preparations

The dosage of iron preparations is calculated on the basis of its elemental iron content. In adults a dose of 50 to 100 mg of elemental iron three times daily is recommended which can be obtained from the following oral dosage forms.

Ferrous sulphate tablets : 300mg three times a day is most effective. Nearly 15% of the oral dose is absorbed from the gastrointestinal tract. The other preparations are Ferrous gluconate and Ferrous fumarate used in the dose of 600 and 500mg respectively three times a day which contain 33% of available iron in tablets.

Ferric ammonium citrate : 1 gm three times a day. Not commonly used.

Reduced iron : This is considered as effective as ferrous sulphate provided it has a small particle size. The usual dose is 500mg three times a day.

Side effects of oral iron preparations are common to all salts. They are upper gastric discomfort, constipation and diarrhea related to iron induced changes in the bacterial flora of the intestine. This is seen more at high doses.

Parenteral iron preparations : When there is low degree of efficiency of oral iron absorption parenteral iron can be used.

Iron dextran injections : This is a complex of ferric hydroxide with dextran in a colloidal solution. It contains 50mg of iron per ml. It is given intramuscularly in an initial dose of 1 to 2ml which can be increased up to 10ml at a time. Side effects are fever, generalized lymphadenopathy, malaise and urticaria.

Other Iron Preparations : Ferrous lactate, Ferrous Gluconate; Ferrous fumarate and Ferrous calcium citrate.

These organic acid salts of Iron, are less apt to produce gostrointestinal irritation.

Administration of Iron : Iron salts should be administered shorthy after meals to reduce gastric irritation. A tolerance may be induced by starting with a small dose and gradually increasing it.

8.1.2. Pernicious Anemia

Most common cause of pernicious anemia is vitamin B_{12} and folic acid deficiency with the manifestation of megaloblastic anemia. Vitamin B_{12} forms a complex with intrinsic factor which is a glycoprotein produced by parietal cells of the stomach. This is absorbed from the small intestine as intrinsic factor-B_{12} complex to be transported to the bone marrow. Once vitamin B_{12} is in circulation it is transported to the tissue by plasma globulin and stored preferentially in the liver. A portion of the stored vitamin is secreted into bile and reabsorbed in the ileum.

Vitamin B_{12} is essential for cell growth and for maintenance of normal myelin. Vitamin B_{12} functions as cobamide coenzyme which is involved in many biochemical processes such as enzymatic conversion of methyl malonyl coenzyme A to succinyl coenzyme A in the body tissues.

It has been observed that methyl malonic acid appears in excess in the urine in patients with pernicious anemia which disappears on vitamin B_{12} treatment.

Dosage forms of vitamin B_{12} : Cyanocobalmine injection : Available in strength of 250, 500, 1000 micro gram per ml. which can be administered intramuscularly. Sensitivity to the injection of vitamin B_{12} by skin test is to be carried out before its administration as it may show anaphylaxis.

Hydroxy cobalamin injection : Available in the strength of 250 and 1000 micro gram per ml for intra muscular injection which may have more sustained effect.

Folic Acid : This is a combination of pteridine p-aminobenzoic acid and glutamic acid or pteroylglutamic acid. It occurs in green vegetables. Deficiency occurs due to malnutrition or by administration of folic acid antagonist like methotrexate, an anticancer agent.

Dosage form of Folic acid : Tablets of folic acid containing 1 to 5mg of the agent for oral administration.

Tablets of Folinic acid which contains 15mg of the agent is used to intercept the action of inhibitors of dihydrotolate reductase like methotrexate but not indicated in folic acid deficiency.

Drug interaction : In large doses it may counteract phenytoin group of drugs used as antiepileptics.

Prevention of thrombosis

The process of intravascular blood clot formation is known as thrombosis. Thrombosis can reduce blood flow to the brain and myocardium which can be fatal. Clotting occurs due to interactions between components of vessel walls and circulating blood platelet and plasma proteins. The simplest biochemical sequence in clotting is as follows :

The soluble protein fibrinogen in plasma is converted to insoluble fibrin by an enzyme thrombin. Thrombin itself is not present as such in normal blood plasma. It is liberated from its precursor prothrombin. Prothrombin is a glycoprotein with a glutamate residue synthesised in the liver in presence of vitamin K. The activation of prothrombin occurs on the blood platelets and phospholipids present on the internal side of platelet membrane which is exposed as a result of collagen induced platelet adhesion. Platelet phospholipids bind to calcium ion which in turn binds to the glutamate region of the prothrombin. An activated zymogen of serine protease known as stuart-prower factor (Factor-x) cleaves the prothrombin to thrombin assisted by another activated proaccelerin accelerator globulin and calcium ion.

Proaccelerin accelerator globulin is one of the clotting factor which also acts on the receptor for the activated stuart-prower factor which binds to prothrombin and converts it to thrombin. Fibrinogen is a plasma protein consisting of six poly peptide chains. The ends of the fibrinogen molecule are highly negatively charged. These negatively charged termini of the fibrinogen molecule contribute to its water solubility but also repulse the termini of the other fibrinogen molecules there by preventing aggregation. Thrombin breaks the peptide linkage. Consequently the repulsive forces between the termini of the fibrinogen vanish and which aggregation takes place to form fibrin polymer clot which traps the red cells, platelets and other components of blood to form the thrombus.

8.2. ANTICOAGULANTS

Chemicals and drugs can act at different points of coagulation to act as anticoagulants and thrombolytics. Chemicals like calcium oxalate, citrate and EDTA prevent blood clotting in vitro. All of them produce their action by virtue of their effect on ionized calcium. However these chemicals are not effective in vivo because ionized levels are sufficiently low to obtain an anticoagulant effect and all the above mentioned chemicals are incompatible with living organism.

8.2.1. Heparin

Heparin is a sterile preparation containing the sodium salt of a complex organic acid present in mammalian tissues having the characteristic property of delaying the clotting of shed blood. It contains not less than 100 Units per mg, calculated with reference to the substance dried to constant weight at 60°C. The potency of a sample of heparin is determined by comparing the concentration necessary to prevent clotting of shed blood, with the concentration of the standard preparation necessary to give the same effect. The standard preparation is a quantity of the dried sodium salt of heparin prepared from the crystallised barium salt of ox heparin. The unit is the specific activity contained in such an amount of the standard preparation as stated in pharmacopoeia. Heparin is a charged molecule that can block clotting both *in vitro* and *in vivo*. The anticoagulant effect of heparin is because of inhibition of several activated clotting factors. In low concentrations heparin increases the activity of antithrombion against activated stuartprower factor and thrombin. So low doses of heparin are used. It is not absorbed from the oral route so it is administered as intravenous injection. The half life of heparin varies from 1 to 2 hours. Heparin is available as injections having 1000 to 40000 units per ml.

100 USP units correpond to about 1mg of heparin. The total daily dose is 500 units per kg body weight. The effect of an over dose can be antagonised by protamine sulphate.

Heparin is contraindicated for concomitent use with aspirin and oral anticoagulants. Heparin is very inert pharmacologically except for its anticoagulant action. It has no significant effect on blood pressure, heart rate and respiration. Adverse effects are bleeding from mucous membrane, long term use may result in osteoporosis. It may show hypersensitivity reactions.

8.2.2. Oral Anticoagulants

These drugs have been derived from coumarin and indanedione molecules. The basic mechanism of action is the inhibition of prothrombin formation and other vitamin K dependent clotting factors such as stuart-prower factor. The coumarin anticoagulants are Dicumarol, Warfarin, Acenocumarol and Phenprocumon. The indandion derivatives are phenindion, and Diphenandion.

All these compounds take time to exihibit their therapeutic effecti in comparison to heparin. This time lag is because the normal prothrombin content of the plasma has to decline before the evidence of deficient prothrombin formation can manifest itself. All the compounds vary in their onset of action and duration because their absorption and metabolism rates are different. Hence all of them have an average initial dose followed by a maintenance dose as the kinetics of the anticoagulant effect depends on inhibited clotting factors. The average daily doses of some coumarin and indandion derivatives with their common side effects are given in the following Table :

Name	Initial dose (mg)	Maintenance dose (mg)	Common side effects
Dicumarol	300	100 to 200	gastrointestinal effects like nausea, flatulence abdominal pain Haemorragic-diasthesis
Warfarin sodium	60	10	
Acenocumarol	15 to 25	2 to 10	
Phenprocoumon	20 to 30	1 to 5	
Phenindione	100 to 200	25 to 50	
Diphenadion	20 to 30	15	

Many factors increase or decrease the response of an oral anticoagulant. Vitamin K deficiency, chronic alcoholism, hyperthyroidism and age vary the response of these drugs. They are protein bound to a maximum extent so displacement from the protein bound state by any other drug will give a higher concentration of the free drug to give rise to drug-drug interaction. Phenylbutazone group of drugs produce such interactions by displacement from the protein bound state. Cimetidine inhibits the metabolism of coumarine anticoagulants. Similarly metronidazole, sulfinpyrazone and trimethoprim. sulphamethoxazole prolong half life of warfarin. So concomitant administration of these group of drugs with oral anticoagulants require readjustment of the doses. Similarly some drugs can reduce the response of oral anticoagulants. Notably the effect of hepatic microsomal inducers, such as barbiturates enhance clearance of oral anticoagulants. Griseofulvin and rifampin decrease the effect of coumarin derivatives. Coumarin also potentiates the effect of tolbutamide and phenytoin.

8.2.3. Antithrombolytic Agents

These drugs are used for prevention and dissolving the blood clot.

Streptokinase : This is a fibrinolytic enzyme used for dissolving blood clot. Streptokinase is administered in a dose of 1-2 million i.u. by intra venous infusion in acute myocardial infarction, deep venous thrombosis and acute arterial occlusion by thrombi.

The agent is contraindicated in cerebral arterial disease and if there is a disease with active bleeding.

Dipyridamol : This agent is a antiplatelet drug. The drug is used in a dose of 400 mg per day for inhibiton of thrombocytic aggregation. It is also a vasodilator and can be used in combination with aspirin in a dose of 75 mg eight hourly. The drug is contraindicated in peptic ulcer and in haemodynamic instability associated with recent myocardial infarction or any other condition.

Aspirin : Aspirin in a dose of 50mg once daily at the same time each day can be administered as prophylaxis in case of increased risk of blood clotting. It inhibits platelet aggregation by blocking the enzyme of the platelet that are responsible for the synthesis of the precursor of prostaglandins. It is contraindicated in persons sensitive to aspirin and peptic ulcer and in platelet disorder.

8.3. DRUGS USED IN HYPERLIPIDEMIA

Antihyperlipidemic agents are indicated for the modification of abnormal serum lipid profile. Abnormal blood lipids have been associated with diseases that arise out of arteriosclerosis, with an increase of blood cholesterol. Alteration in lipid metabolism leads to hyperlipidemic state. A normal blood sample has the following lipid profile.

Total cholesterol lies in the range of 150 to 240mg per 100ml of the blood. High level of serum cholesterol usually shows an increase in concentration of low density lipoprotein cholesterol (LDLC) which accounts for 60 to 70% of the total blood cholesterol.

The normal value of LDLC is 150mg per 100ml of blood.

The other factor which is important in the determination of hyperlipidemia is the concentration of high density lipoprotein cholesterol (HDLC). This is present in blood in a range of 38 to 64mg per 100 ml of the blood.

The ratio of LDLC to HDLC should be less than 3 in normal individuals. Any value above this warrants attention.

Most of the hypercholesterolemic conditions are due to the defect in receptor mediated catabolism of LDL cholesterol. Secondary lipoprotein cholesterol abnormalities are due to the defect in receptor mediated catabolism of LDL cholesterol.

Secondary lipoprotain cholesterol abnormilities are associated with endocrine disorders such as diabetes mellitus, hyperthyroidism, obesity and kidney diseases. Drugs can also induce change in the lipid profile, such as thiazide diuretics may lower HDLC and may raise triglycerides and LDLC levels in blood. There are a number of different types of drugs used in lowering blood cholesterol.

Nicotinic acid (Nicin) : This drug depresses the synthesis of very low density lipoproteins. Nicin is used in the dose of 1gm daily in combination with fish oil. 300 to 600mg capsules produce lowering of triglycerides and LDLC. It is used in the therapy of hyperlipidemia.

Nicin can cause flushed skin, itching, hyperuricemia and decreased glucose tolerance.

Drobucol : This is structurally related to tochopherol used in the dose of 500mg twice daily. This drug lowers both LDLC and HDLC levels. The side effects are diarrhea, dyspepsia and skin rash.

Ion exchange resins : *Cholestyramine* is a chloride salt of basic anion exchange resin. This agent being insoluble in water and is unaffacted by digestive enzymes remains unabsorbed during the passage through the intestine. It binds to the bile salts and is excreted in the stool. This process reduces the normal bile acid, so the net result is an increase of hepatic conversion of cholesterol into bile acid which is excreted with the resin.

8 to 24 gm with a suitable liquid is given in 1 to 3 divided doses before meals. Common side effects are dyspepsia, constipation, nausea and abdominal pain. It retards the absorption of many drugs. The other drug is Colestipol which is a copolymer of diethyl enetriamine and chloroepoxypropane.

It is administered in a dose of 5 to 30gm in suitable suspenson daily before meals. The side effects are common to cholestyramine.

9

HORMONES AND RELATED DRUGS

The hormones are products of specialized tissues known as endocrine glands that partcipate in many metabolic processes. The hormones vary in their structure and chemically they may be relatively simple organic compounds to complex polypeptides and proteins. In addition to the naturally occuring hormones synthetic substitutes are also used with some advantages over the naturally occuring ones. Hermones find their use in substitution therapy in endocrine deficiencies and also to induce pharmacological actions related to their normal functions. The present section deals with some hormones and their congeners that act on certain endocrine glands to modify their secretory activity and affect the end organs to modify their functions.

9.1. GLUCOCORTICOIDS AND RELATED DRUGS

The adrenal cortex secrete glucocorticoids that affect carbohydrate and protein metabolism. Hydrocortisone in the form of cortisol sodium succinate, an endogenous glucocorticoid is given as intravenous injection as replacement therapy for adrenal insufficiency of acute nature. The other endogenous glucocorticoids are cortisone and corticosterone. Cortisone acetate is used for chronic adrenal insufficiency.

Physiological functions of glucocorticoids are to increase liver glycogen store, increase gluconeogenesis, lipolysis, maintain skeletal muscle function and increase hemoglobin synthesis.

However pharmacotherapeutic effect can result if administered in appropriate doses like anti inflammatory and antiallergic effects. Steroids can cause suppression of leucocyte migration and reduce the activity of fibroblast which are increased at the site of chronic inflammation. They can counteract histamine release by affecting the capillary permeability and also supress the immune response by inhibiting antibody synthesis.

Mechanism of action : Once the steroids cross the cell membrane they bind to a receptor with the formation of steroid receptor complex in the cell nucleus and then bind to the chromatin or the chromosomal substance. This chromatin-steroid-receptor complex stimulates the formation of messenger RNA which in turn stimulates the synthesis of enzymes that control the limiting reactions that account for the actions of corticosteroids.

Glucocorticoids have multiple therapeutic uses :

1. Relacement therapy in Addisons disease which is due to primary adrenal insufficiency. Also used in hypopituitarism.

2. Immunosuppression-Collagen disease such as systemic lupus erythematosus which denotes widespread inflammatory changes in the connective tissue affecting the skin, joints, lungs etc. Also in rheumatoid arthritis and ankylosing spondylitis.

3. Suppression of inflammatory oedema of acute polyneuritis and cholestatic jaundice.

4. Acute illnesses-Anaphlaxis, septicemia, status asthmaticus, lymphatic leukemia, and acute exfoliative dermatitis.

5. Local use-Allergic eye conditions and eczema. Glucocorticoids that are therapeutically used can be divided into two groups

   (a) *Glucocorticoids with minerolocorticoid activity* such as *Hydrocortisone and Cortisone.* Show sodium, phosphate, bicarbonate retention with the reduction of serum potassium.

   (b) *Glucocorticoids without mineralo-corticoid activity are Prednisone, Prednisolone. Betamethasone. Beclome-thasone, Dexamethasone* and *Methylprednisolone.*

All the above agents are absorbed from the oral route and 90% of the drugs get plasma protein bound. They are metabolised by the liver and excreted by kidney as conjugates. Predinisolone and the other glucocorticoids inhibit phospholipase in a number of tissues thereby blocking all eicosanoid formation in these tissues. Thus prednisolone group of drugs block the synthesis of prostaglandins, leukotrienes and thromboxanes which probably explains their potent antiinflammatory effect. Moreover, leukotrienes play a role in hypersensitivity reactions so their suppression explains the efficacy of conticosteroids in allergic disorders.

Above mentioned group of agents can be classified according to their duration of action :

(a) Short acting with less than 12 hours of duration of action are hydrocortisone and cortisone.

(b) Intermediate acting having a duration from 13 to 24 hours are prednisolone, prednisone, methylprednisolone and triamcinolone. All are more potent than hydrocortisone with reference to anti-inflammatory action and show very little sodium retention properties in comparison to hydrocortisone.

(c) Long acting with more than 24 hours of action are betamethasone and dexamethasone, have maximum anti inflammatory potency with minimum sodium retention. Beclomethasone is available in inhalation dosage form and can be used in bronchial asthma.

Adverse effects of corticosteroids : Prolonged therapy can suppress pituitary and adrenal functions. It can increase susceptibility to infections on prolonged use. There can be peptic ulceration as a result of altered defence mechanism of gastric mucosal wall. It inhibits osteoblast, the cell associated with bone production and so it can lead to osteoporosis.

In children it can arrest growth as it also inhibits DNA synthesis and cell division.

Contraindications : Corticosteroids are contraindicated in tuberculosis, peptic ulcer, renal dysfuction, osteoporosis. Withdrawl of the drug should be gradual.

9.2. ORAL CONTRACEPTIVES

Hormonal oral contraceptives are the group of preparations that primarily inhibit ovulation so that conception cannot occur. Ovulation is under the control of follicle stimulating hormone (FSH) and lutenizing hormone (LH) which are released from anterior pitutary gland. All this happens periodically under the influence of gonadotropin released by hypothalamus which affects the function of anterior pitutary gland, i.e. release of FSH and LH.

Mode of action of hormonal oral contraceptives : The role of estrogen has an important bearing on the mode of action of hormonal oral contraceptives. It has been observed that in the first five days of menstural cycle the blood level of estrogen rises. During this period follicles that are pouch like depressions or cavities develop in the ovary under the influence of FSH. In the next phase estrogen level decreases in the blood because of less secretion. On about 14th day folicles rupture with occurance of ovulation and also corpus luteum is formed. Corpus luteum is a fibrous tissue that is formed soon after ovulation when pregnancy does not supervene. After 14th day the corpus luteum formed in the previous sequence secretes progesterone and estrogen and the blood level of these two hormones remain elevated till the corpus luteum regresses.

This is the reason why oral contraceptive pills contain estrogen and progesterone in such concentrations which can suppress the mid cycle stimulation of LH and FSH which triggers ovulation.

Combination Pills

Commonly used pills contain Ethinyl estradiol or mestranol for estrogenic activity and Norethindrone, Ethynodrel or Norethynodrel for progesterone activity. Different combination pills may contain one of the above mentioned estrogenic compound and progesterone. Combination pills have a dose of both estrogen and a progestin and their, administration starts on day 5 and continued for 12 to 16 days till day 25.

Contraindication of combination pills : Thrombotic disorders, cerebrovascular and cardiovascular disorders, and impaired liver function. Control of fertility can be done with other dosage preparations such as minipill and the triphasic pills.

Minipill : This contains only progestin delivered in a very low dose e.g. about 35 to 70 µg of progesterone a day from a suitable dosage form. A drug delivery system particularly of the synthetic polymer variety has found wide spread application in the area of contraception. Levonorgestrel tablet containing 30 µg produces its effect by thickening the consistency of cervical mucous thereby providing a barrier to the sperm and control and fertility.

Triphasic Pills

The combination pills show an adverse effect in some women known as break through bleeding in the form of irregular vaginal bleeding when combination pills are first started. To minimize this effect triphasic pills have been developed which provide one estrogen dose with varying progesterone doses in order to reflect the changing progesterone levels during the follicular, ovulatory and luteinizing phases of the menstural cycle.

Triphasic pills can have a fixed dose of ethinyloestradiol 35 µg and varying progestin viz. norethindrone in the strength of 0.5 mg in the first seven days then 0.75 mg in the next seven days and lastly 1 mg dose for the next seven days. Other uses of combination pills are in the control and reduction of ovarian and endrometrial cancer, benign fibrocystic breast disease and ovarian cysts. It can also be used in menorrhagia.

Estrogen : Female sex hormone estrogen is available as conjugated estrogen tablets of strength 1.5 mg Estradiol valerate in the form of injection. Estriol succinate tablets in the strength of 2 mg and Stilbestrol tablets in the strength of 1 mg. Estrogen is used in hypogonadal disorders such as hypopituitarism. It increases circulating renin and angiotensin and so it can cause hypertension.

Clomiphen : Clomiphen citrate tablets in a dose of 50 mg daily can be used for infertility. It produces a surge in FSH and induces ovulation. It can cause multiple pregnancy.

9.3. INSULIN AND ORAL HYPOGLYCIMIC DRUGS

Insulin and oral hypoglycemic agents are used in the treatment of diabetes mellitus. Dlabetes can be of adult onset type or juvenile diabetes. In adult onset diabetes only half of the beta cells that secrete insulin from the pancreas may remain active where as in the other form of diabetes the panereas is non-functional. The lack of insulin results in a peripheral underutilization and a hepatic overproduction of glucose. This is reflected as hyperglycemia, as a net result we find a rise in the fasting blood sugar level of the individual. Whenever the fasting blood sugar level is more than 100mg per 100ml of blood it requires attention because the normal range of fasting blood sugar lies between 60 to 100 mg glucose per 100ml.

The physiological function of insulin is to facilitate the entry of glucose into the cell for further metabolism and utilization.

It has been observed that diabetes not only involves the deficiency of insulin but sometimes an excess of certain other hormones such as the growth hormone, glucocorticoids and glucagon can give rise to hyperglycemia. Insulin synthesis is controlled by an enzymatic process and stored in granules which are released by the the process of exocytosis. Oral glucose, fatty acids, and ketone bodies can stimulate insulin secretion, Gastrointestinal hormone like pancreozymin, gastrin and secretin can also stimulate insulin secretion.

Besides these there can be an autonomic control of insulin secretion because it has been observed that beta agonists increase insulin secretion by increasing cyclic AMP which together with calcium ion activates the insulin release. Insulin circulates in blood as free hormone and is degraded by the proteolytic enzyme in the liver.

Insulin deficiency reduces the rate of transport of glucose across the cell membrane. Besides hyperglycemia there can be hyperlipemia, ketonemia and acidosis in insulin deficiency.

Action of insulin is at the cell surface where the hormone interacts with a specific receptor to facilitate the transport of glucose into the cell. Insulin occurs as monomer, a dimer or in the hexamer form. The hexamer has three dimers coordinated by a zinc molecule and is stored in the beta cells of the pancreas. The amino acid sequence of insulin varies from species to species.

Preparations of Insulin

Injection of Insulin is a sterile solution of the specific antidiabetic principle of the mammalian pancreas containing 20, 40 or 80 units per ml. The potency of an injection of insulin is determined by biological assay by comparing the hypoglycemic effect it produces with that produced by a standard preparation of insulin under specified conditions of the assay technique. The standard preparation is a quantity of pure, dry, crystalline insulin as specified in a pharmacopoeia and is expressed in units per ml.

There are various types of insulin which differ in their onset of action and duration.

(a) **Soluble insulin** is short acting having approximately a duration of effect of 6 to 8 hours. It is prepared in a suitable buffer with zinc. It is administered subcutaneously or intravenously and can give a rapid control of diabetic ketoacidosis. The dose is determined in accordance with the needs of the patient.

(b) **Insulin protamine zinc injection :** It is an insoluble complex formed by insulin with protamine. Addition of basic protein protamine to crystalline zinc insulin causes the formation of large crystals of insoluble protamine zinc insulin. When it is injected it serves as a tissue depot producing slow absorption into blood. The duration of action of this preparation is 24 to 36 hours.

(c) **Lente insulin :** Insulin zinc lente is a preparation of a mixture of 3 parts of amorphous insulin zinc suspension and 7 parts of crystalline insulin zinc suspension. The onset and duration of effect varies with the physical state and zinc concentration and pH.

(d) **Ultra lente insulin:** This is a crystalline form with high zinc content with a duration of action which may vary between 24 to 36 hours.

Drug interactions : Insulin requirement may increase with concomitant use of corticosteroids, oral contraceptives, thyroid hormones, growth hormones and thiazide diuretics. Similarly it may decrease by concomitant use of beta blockers, MAO inhibitors, anticoagulants and salicylates.

Human Insulin : This is a semi synthetic product produced by recombinant DNA techniques. It may have different onset of action and duration than the preparations obtained from the animal source. The advantage of human insulin is that insulin allergy and fat hypertrophy occurs less frequently . It is possible that anti-insulin antibody formation is slightly less with the human hormone. Its antigenic response for hypersensitivity reactions is much less than bovine, pork or highly purified pork insulin but has no other added advantage.

Oral Hypoglycemic Drugs

The commonly used drugs belonging to this group are sulphonylureas. These drugs act by stimulating release of insulin from the beta cells of the pancreas.

They have the capacity to increase the number of insulin receptors in the target tissue thereby enhancing insulin mediated glucose disposal. Some of the oral hypoglycemic drugs used in the treatment of maturity onst diabetes such as biguanides like *phenformin* lower the blood glucose by inhibiting gluconeogenesis in the liver although it may also increase the number of insulin receptors in some tissues. It is used in combination with sulphonylureas to control diabetes if it is not controlled by a single drug.

Phenformin can produce lactic acidosis and so it is not used routinely as the drug of choice. The main sulphonylurea derivatives used as oral hypoglycemic drugs are: *Tolbutamide, Chlorpropamide, Acetohexamide, Tolazamide, Glyburide and Clipizide.* All of them stimulate insulin secretion, induce activity of peripheral insulin receptors and also may reduce the secretion of glucagon, the insulin inhibitor. *Tolbutamide :* It is a short acting agent. The onset of action is 30 minutes, the effect remaining from six to twelve hours. It is metabolized by liver and excreted by kidney. *Chlorpropamide :* It is rapidly absorbed with a duration of action of 60 hours as it is bound to plasma proteins to a large extent. It is metabolized slowly by liver and the drug is also excreted unchaged in the urine. A dose of 100 to 500mg a day can produce its effect for 60 hours.

Acetohexamide : It has a rapid onset of action. Acetohexamide shows its peak effect in 3hours and the action lasts for 12 to 24 hours. the daily dose of the drug lies between 250 to 1500 mg once or twice a day this being determind according to the patients requirement. Its metabolite, hydroxyhexamide is responsible for its activity. The drug is mainly excreted via the kidney.

Tolazamide : This drug shows hypoglycemic action in a daily dose which lies between 100 to 1000 mg to be given once or twice a day. It is slowly absorbed with a duration of action of 24 hours. It has also a metabolite that has weaker hypoglycemic effect than the parent drug. It is excreted by the kidney.

Glyburide and Glipizide : These two drugs show their effect in very small doses in comparison to other oral hypoglycemics. The duration of action for both of them is 24 hours.

The daily dose of glyburide is 1.25 to 20 mg to be given once or twice a day as per the patients requirement.

The dose of glipizide is between 2.5 to 40mg for the control of diabetes. *Adverse effect* of sulphonylureas are minimum but hepatic and renal insufficiency can cause longer duration of action because all of them are metabolized and excreted by liver and kidneys. Inappropriate secretion of antidiuretic hormone has also been observed with sulphonylureas.The other side effects are epigastric pain and skin rash and blood dycrasias have also been reported.

Drug interactions with sulphonylureas are encountered because of competitive plasma protein binding. So adjustment of dose is required for drugs which are concomitantly administered that may compete for protein binding. The examples of such drugs are oxyphenbutazone, oral coumarin anticoagulants, sulpha drugs, and chloramphenicol. Hypoglycemic effects are reduced by corticosteroids, and thiazide diuretics.

9.4. THYROID HORMONES AND ANTITHYROID DRUGS

Thyroid gland is associated with the secretion of L-Thyroxin (T_4) and 3,5,3 triiodo-L-Thyronine (T_3). A quantitive alteration of hormone secretion or enlargement of the thyroid or both are manifested in the disease state of the thyroid gland. Thyroid function test is done by thyroid radio active iodine uptake. This can also be carried out by estimation of hormone concentration. The normal range of T_4 is 5 to 12 ug per 100ml and T_3 values range between 70 to 190 ng per 100ml of blood.

Thyroid hormones regulate growth and development of the body. They accelerate glucose utilization by increasing the basal metabolic rate. Lipolytic reaction is enhanced so plasma cholesterol may decrease. It can also stimulate the cardio-vascular system causing palpitation which can be treated with a beta blocking agent like propranolol.

Myxedema or hypothyroidism requires thyroid hormone therapy. Preparations used in hormone therapy are thyroid tablets.

Thyroid tablets : It contains dry extract of thyroid obtained from the thyroid glands of oxen, sheep, or pigs. It contains 0.1 percent of iodine as thyroxine and mixed with sufficient quantity of lactose to produce a powder of the required strength. The dose of each tablet is 30mg to be given as per requirement. Thyroid tablets contain Thyroglobulin as purified thyroid extract having L-thyroxin and L-triiodothyronin. The drug is contraindicated in cardiovascular disease. Thyroid deficiency can also be treated with Thyroxine sodium tablets. The dose is 0.05 to 0.2mg per day for hypothyroidism, myxoedema & cretinism. Myxoedema is an abnormal skin condition with deposits of mucin associated with hypothyroidism. Cretinism is the arrested physical and mental development due to congenital lack of thyroid secretion. The drug is contraindicated in adrenal insufficiency and lactation, and thyrotoxicosis.

Anti Throid Drugs

Thyroid inhibitors are used when the body is exposed to an excess of thyroid hormone leading to thyrotoxicosis, a syndrome that can originate in a variety of ways including over production of the thyroid hormone. Anti thyroid drugs are *propyl-thiouracil* and *Methimazole*. The mode of action of both the drugs are inhibition of iodine incorporation in the biosynthesis of the hormone. Propylthiouracil inhibits conversion of T_4 to T_3 and it has a shorter half life than methimazole.

Adverse effects of both drugs are marked decrease in the number of granulocytes and leucopenia. Joint pain and depigmentation of hair can also occur. The other thyroid inhibitors like iodides in high concentration can suppress the thyroid.

Radioactive iodine given in sufficient amount to suppress the thyroid can produce cytotoxic effect due to the ionizing radiation.

10

LOCAL ANAESTHETICS

Pressure on the nerve trunks or paralysing the sensory nerve fibers with a drug or the application of hypothermia can induce local anaesthesia. Application of hypothermia by means of a spray of *Ethyl chloride* is a convenient method of producing local anaesthesia of small area of skin for a few seconds. However lasting effect cannot be produced because prolonged freezing kills the tissue. Super cooling is used in patients in whom an injured limb requires amputation. Many drugs can paralyse nerve endings. However, they also injure the surrounding tissue, e.g. a 5 percent solution of phenol produces partial anaesthesia without any specific action on nerve ending and phenol destroys the surface tissue of the exposed sensory nerve endings.

Clove oil : The active ingredient in clove oil is *Eugenol, a* phenolic substance which is useful in relieving tooth ache. Phenols when applied to the surface of a tooth cavity anesthetise any sensitive dentine that is exposed.

CLASSIFICATION OF LOCAL ANAESTHETICS

Local anaesthetics are divided into two groups :

    (a) Water soluble

    (b) Water insoluble

      The water soluble agents are usually tertiary amino esters of an aromatic acid e.g. procaine, amethocain, butacaine and cocaine. The other water soluble local anaesthetics are substituted amides like dibucaine (cinchocaine) and lignocaine (lidocaine). The water insoluble local anaesthetics are esters of aminobenzoic acid e.g. ethyl amino benzoate (benzocaine) and butyl amino benzoate (butesin). These drugs are used as ointments or dusting powders owing to their low solubiity.

MODE OF ACTION OF LOCAL ANAESTHETICS

Local anaesthetic drugs block nerve conduction by a reversible inactivation of the mechanism responsible for sodium transport. The conduction of an impulse along a nerve depends on a complex series of changes in permeability of the nerve membrane to sodium and potassium ions. The sodium transport mechanism can readily be deranged by drugs and when this occurs conduction of the nerve impulse is blocked. It has been observed that local anaesthetics paralyse sensory nerve fibres before motor fibers. This is not due to a specific affinity for sensory fibres but can be accounted for by the smaller size of these fibres which allows a more rapid penetration by the local anaesthetic drugs.

INDUCTION OF LOCAL ANAESTHESIA

Local anaesthesia can be induced in a number of ways :

1. **Surface anaesthesia :** The drug is applied directly to the skin or mucous membrane to produce a paralyzing effect due to blockade of the afferent nerve ends. Local anaesthetics that readily penetrate mucous membranes are widely used for producing surface anaesthesia in the eye, nose, and throat.

2. **Infiltration anaesthesia :** The anaesthetic diluted in normal saline is injected into the tissue through a fine hypodermic needle, the surrounding structure becomes swollen and edematous, fit for surgical procedure.

3. **Conduction anaesthesia :** This consists in injecting a local anaesthetic into the immediate neighborhood of the nerve supplying the part to be operated on.

4. **Regional anaesthesia :** This designates procedures in which the local anaesthetic is applied along the course of a nerve for example spinal anaesthesia. In this the agent is passed into the spinal canal between the laminae of the

lumber vertebrae, the anesthetic dissolved in a small amount of spinal fluid is introduced into the subarachnoid space. Spinal and other forms of regional anaesthesia have a number of advantages over general anaesthesia.

INDIVIDUAL LOCAL ANAESTHETICS

Cocaine

It is an alkaloid obtained from the leaves of the Coca tree (Erythroxylon coca). In addition to its local action in paralyzing the sensory nerve, cocaine also exerts important systemic effects. The following are the systemic effects. It increases the blood pressure, accelerates pulse rate, accelerates respiration, dilates the pupil, elevates body temperature and blood sugar. All these actions are similar to the actions that follow stimulation of the adrenergic nerves. However these effects are not mediated through peripheral mechanism but are of central origin because in animal experiments it can be shown that transecting the spinal cord will abolish these effects. Cocaine is a CNS stimulant. It causes wakefulness, motor excitement and increases the power of endurance to fatigue. All these properties lead to drug abuse and addiction.

Procaine

It is a synthetic substitute of cocaine but is less toxic than cocaine. The safety of the drug depends upon its slow absorption because the liver can metabolize it rapidly. It is non irritant and is used for infiltration and spinal anesthesia. Procaine can sensitize the skin to cause procaine dermatitis. *Toxic effects* are convulsions followed by respiratory paralysis and it can cause sudden fall in blood pressure.

Lignocaine (Lidocaine, Xylocaine)

Lignocaine is about two and half times as active as procaine. It is rapidly absorbed from the mucous membrane and is used for surface and infiltration anaesthesia. It is also an effective topical anesthetic. Lignocaine jelly prepared with carboxymethyl cellulose is used in all types of urethral manipulation and catheterisation. *Toxic effects* are dizziness, drowsiness, muscle twitching, bradycardia and hypotension.

11

BIOLOGICAL ASSAY

The estimation of the active principle in a drug done by an approved biological method which is intended to provide guarantee of the therapeutic efficacy is referred as biological assay. Biological assays and tests are prescribed for those drugs whose potency cannot be adequately determined by chemical or physical means. In biological assay the potency of a drug is determined by means of a biological indicator. The biological reaction is not always identical because many conditions may alter the extent to which an animal reacts to a drug, so every precaution must be taken to keep the conditions uniform in performing these tests.

To minimize biological variation animals must be, as far as possible, of the same weight and age. The test must be done upon a series of animals sufficiently large to eliminate the variations that cannot be controlled. In order to overcome the variation between conditions it is necessary to compare the unknown preparation with a standard preparation.

These reference standards are maintained by the pharmacopeial authorities. If the potency of a drug is expressed in units, then the unit is defined as a definite weight of the standard preparation required to produce a certain effect specific to the drug under test. Due to the variations in the biological responses used in bioassay, the results of each assay must be subjected to statistical analysis.

METHODS OF BIOLOGICAL ASSAY

The indicators used in biological assay are as follows :

(a) Assay depending upon the measurement of effective dose for each animal.

(b) Assay depending upon quantal effect.

(c) Assay depending upon measured graded dose response.

(a) Measurement of the effective dose for each animal is the basis for this assay. The determination of the end point in each case is noted from a specific pharmacological effect of the drug e.g. in the assay of digitalis in guinea pigs the stopping of the heart reveals the individual lethal dose. Similarly in the assay of tubocurarine in rabbits the head drop indicating complete relaxation of the neck muscle is taken to be the end point. Thus the amount of each drug required for reaching the end point is determined to obtain an estimate of potency ratio of a given preparation to the standard preparation.

In this assay there are two groups of estimates of individual effective dose. One depicting the results of the standard preparation and the other that of the unknown preparation of the same drug. For calculation, each estimate obtained from the end point in the respective individual animal is converted to a logarithm and the mean is calculated with its standard deviation. The ratio of the potency is obtained from the antilogerathim of the mean differences.

(b) **Quantal or all or none assay :** In this assay the percentage of positive effects are measured. Each animal is categorised as responding or non responding according to a prior decided criterion of response. For example in the assay of digitalis with frogs or that of insulin with mice, death or hypoglycemic convulsant effect respectively may be noted as either occuring or not occuring in each animal and the result depends on the number of animals in which it occurs. Such assays are called quantal or all or none because we obtain a percentage of animals showing a positive response at each dose level.

The percentage of animals giving a positive response to each dose is then converted into a probit, which is taken as a measure of the effect.

The dose should be chosen so that the percentage effect is never 0 or 100.

(c) **Graded dose response assay :** Graded dose response assay is based on the proportionate increase in an observed response with an increment in a dose of a drug. Here the size or speed of the reaction is measured at each of two or more dose levels. A suitable function of the response, e.g. contraction of the smooth muscle preparation in the assay of histamine can be plotted as a straight line against the dose or its logarithm. The log-dose response curve is plotted by using at least 4 submaximal concentrations of a known preparation. The concentration of the unknown is then read from the graph, provided the unknown response lies on the linear portion of the dose response curve.

In the other alternative method for the graded dose response assay, the potency may be estimated as the ratio between the two doses of the preparation to be tested to that between the two doses of the standard preparation. In this assay the ratio between two doses of the preparation being tested should be the same as that between two doses of the standard preparation, and this ratio should be kept constant throughout the assay.

The two doses of standard preparation and the two doses of the preparation under test should be given in a random order and at least four responses to each should be recorded. However, in stead of complete randomising., the order of administration is designed in such a manner that it permits the elimination of the effect of changes in the sensitivity of the tissue preparation. The dose should be added at regular intervals of three to five minutes depending upon the rate of recovery of the muscle. All the responses are measured and the result of the assay is calculated by standard statistical methods.

12

DRUG INTERACTION AND
ADVERSE DRUG REACTIONS

DRUG INTERACTION

Interactions between drugs can take place when two or more agents are administered concomitantly. This may lead to altered pharmacological or therapeutic effects of the drugs under consideration. The changes due to such interactions could be either a decrease in the desired effect, increase in unwanted effect, increased plasma levels of the free drug or prolongation of half life of the drug.

There are two main types of interactions between drugs;

　　　(i) Pharmacodynamic interactions.
　　　(ii) Pharmacokinetic interactions.

12.1 PHARMACODYNAMIC INTERACTIONS

Pharmacodyanic interactions are those in which the responsiveness of the target organ or receptor or the physiological system is modified by concomitant administration of the second agent.

Thus there can be physiological antagonism or change in the intra or extra cellular environment e.g. hypokalemia induced by diuretics can cause digitalis toxicity. Another type of pharmacodynamic interaction is chemical inactivation e.g. protamine heparin binding induces neutralization of heparin's action. Pharmacodynamic interaction can also result because an agent may enhance the action of another drug through different mechanisms e.g. alcohol enhances the CNS depression of tranquilizers and morphine like drugs. Similarly a non-steroidal anti inflammatory agent like indomethacin antagonizes the action of beta blockers, diuretics and other drugs. However, no such actions are seen with aspirin.

12.2. PHARMACOKINETIC INTERACTIONS AND DRUG INCOMPATIBILITY

Drug incompatibility of ascorbic acid, ampicillin, or chlorpromazine with dextran solutions (I.V. fluids) occurs either because of drug breakdown or chemical complex formation. Similar inactivation can occur because of interaction between heparin and tetracycline, gentamycin, methicillin and kanamycin. Tetracycline combines with cations like calcium present in milk and some antacids or aluminum present in antacids to form insoluble complexes which are not absorbed and give poor tetracycline blood levels. Pharmacokinetic interactions can cause either diminished or increased systemic delivery of drugs.

Diminished drug delivery :   This can occur because of the folowing reasons.

12.2.1. Impaired Gastro Intestinal Absorption

Cholestyramine, an ion exchange resin used for the treatment of hyperlipidemia binds to drugs like thyroxin and cardiac glycosides and blocks their absorption. Similar effects can be shown by antacids and kaolin-pectin which can hinder the absorption of tetracycline and digoxin respectively. Impaired absorption of drugs results in reduction of the total amount of drug absorbed, with reduced area under the plasma level curve. Also the peak plasma concentrations are reduced and steady state concentration of the drugs that are involved in such interaction are lowered.

12.2.2. Induction of Hepatic Drug Metabolizing Enzymes

The initial step in metabolism of many drugs is excecuted by a group of mixed function oxidase enzyme systems present in the endoplasmic reticulum (cytochrome P_{450} oxidase). The product of these reactions are water soluble in nature so they are readily excreted by the kidney. All barbiturates increase mixed function oxidase isoenzyme activity. Mixed function oxidases are also induced by rifampin, phenytoin and chronic alcohol ingestion.

Therefore these enzyme inducers lower plasma levels of drugs like digitoxin, quinidine, cyclosporine, prednisolone, oral contraceptive steroids and meteronidazole and have obvious therapeutic significance.

12.2.3. Inhibition of Cellular Uptake or Binding

Tricyclic antidepressants are potent inhibitors of noradrenaline reuptake. Therefore concomitant administration of amitriptyline group of tricyclic antidepressants abolish antihypertensive effect of guanethidine group of adrenergic neurone blockers. Such an effect can also be considered as pharmacodynamic interaction. Similarly, ephedrine may also antagonize the effect of guanethidine probably by both inhibition of uptake and displacement from the neurone.

Increased drug delivery : This may occur due to followikng reasons :

12.2.4. Competitive Protein Binding

Drug interactions affect the distribution of drugs because of *competitive plasma protein binding*. Displacement of plasma protein bound drug can result in changes in pharmacological effects due to increased plasma level of the free drug. Drugs can sometimes compete for plasma protein binding site. This effect often releases more free drug and thus enhances its pharmacological effects, especially when over 90% of the drug is protein bound. In the following Table 12.1 some drug interactions due to drug displacement has been indicated.

Table 12.1

Strongly bound drug	Drug displaced	Effect of interaction
Oxyphenbutazone Phenylbutazone Clofibrate	Coumarine (warfarin)	Haemorrhage due to over inhibition of prothrombin synthesis in liver.
Dicoumarol Saliylates Phenylbutazone	Sulphonamides	Enhanced sulphonamide activity
Salicylates Sulphonamides	Methotrexate	Increased Methotrexate toxicity.

12.2.5. Inhibition of Drug Metabolism

Inhibition of drug metabolism leads to a rduced drug clearance causing prolonged half life and accumulation. This excessive accumulation due to inhibited metabolism can lead to adverse effects. For example oxidative metabolism of warfarin, nifedipine lidocaine, quinidine, theophyllin and phenytoin can be inhibited by potent inhibitors like organophosphorous insecticides, carbon monoxide and H_2 antagonist like cimetidine. However, ranitidine and famotidine are less inhibitors of oxidative metabolism.

Erythromycin is known to inhibit the metabolism of cyclosporine, warfarin and theophyllin. The inhibition of these drugs be erythromycin is dependent on its blood concentration. Biotransformation of many drugs may be hindered due to presence of other drugs e.g. isoniazide by phenytoin, phenyl butazone by tolbutamide and cyclosporine clearance in presence of prednisolone. Such complications can be controlled by drug blood level monitoring and changing dose schedule.

12.2.6. Inhibition of Renal Elimination

This factor can cause increased drug concentration in the blood e.g. renal tubular secretion contributes substantially to the elimination of penicillin which is inhibited by probenecid, an uricosuric agent. Similarly probenecid, salicylates and methotrexate competitively inhibit the renal tubular transport system causing excessive accummulation of these agents. Decreased clearance of drugs by different mechanisms may also occur e.g. the concentration of digoxin and digitoxin in blood are elevated by quinidine due to inhibition of renal elimination. So there may be increase in cardiac arrhythmia if quinidine is administered concomitantly with the glycosides.

Similarly cyclosporin and verapamil are also known to inhibit the clearance of digoxin which can attribute toits toxic manifestations. The urinary pH influences the elimination of drugs which are weakly acidic or basic in nature because for passive reabsorption, they should be in unionized state. This factor can be of importance in the treatment of an overdose of aspirin or amphetamine like drugs. Alkalinizers like sodium bicarbonate will increase the excretion of weak acidic drugs. Similarly, acidification of the urine can be achieved by administration of ammonium chloride to increase the elimination of a weak basic drug.

12.3. ADVERSE DRUG REACTION

All drugs are coupled with inescapable untoward effects. The magnitude of the adverse reaction is greater especially when drugs are taken by mother during pregnancy and lactation. The known pharmacological actions of any agent can be exaggerated for a number of reasons. However this can be predicted and controlled. In such cases *drug monitoring* can be useful to control the exaggerated pharmacological effects by modification of the doses.

Besides giving an idea whether the therapeutic level is maintained, drug monitoring also helps to assess drug toxicity and patient compliance. In the following table examples have been drawn for some drugs indicating the importance of drug monitoting by determination of plasma concentrations of drugs druring therapy.

12.3.1 Therapeutic Toxic Concentration of Some Drugs

Table 12.2

Drug	Blood concentration for therapeutic	Concentration which manifest Toxic effects	Category
Digoxin	0.8 ngper ml	2.0 ng per ml	Cardiac glycoside.
Digitoxin	12 ng per ml	30 ng per ml	Cardic glycoside
Phenytoin	10 up per ml	20 ug per ml	Antiepliptic
Ethosuximide	40 up per ml	100 ug per ml	Antiepliptic
Lithium	0.5 meq per litre	1.3 meq per litre	Antipsychotic
Lidocain	1.5 ug per ml	5 ug per ml	Antiarrhythmic
procainamide	4 ug per ml	10 ug per ml	Antiarrhythmic
Quinidine	2.5 ug per ml	6 ug per ml	Antiarrhythmic
Theophylline	8 up per ml	20 up per ml	Bronchodilator

Errors in self administration of a prescribed drug can also give rise to adverse effects by not folowing the directions for administration of the drug.

12.3.2 Toxic Effects of a Drug Unrelated to its Pharmacological Actions

These are :

A. Cytotoxicity

B. Abnormal immune response

C. Disturbances in the metabolic functions.

12.3.2.1 Cytotoxic reations : The mechanism of such reactions can be understod from the mode of action of some chemical agents. Carcinogens such as alkylating agents directly combine with the DNA to from irreversible complex through a covalent bond. Such covalent binding occurs usually after metabolic activation of the agent to reactive metabolites. This usually occurs in the microsomal mixed function oxidase system of the hepatic enzymes.

These reactive metabolites may covalently bind to the tissue macromolecules causing tissue damage.

Hepatoxicity of isoniazide can be sited as an example of such an adverse reaction unrelated to its therapeutic effect.

Isoniazide is mainly metabolized by acetylation to acetylisoniazide which on further hydrolysis produces acetylhydrazine. Further metabolism of acetyl hydrazine by mixed function oxidase system liberates reactive metabolites that covalently bind to hepatic macromolecule causing hepatic necrosis. Thus drugs that increase the activity of the mixed function oxidase system e.g. phenobarbital when given together with isoniazide can cause liver damage. Similar explanation holds good for hepatic necrosis from overdose of paracetamol. Normally these metabolites are removed by hepatic glutation. When glutation is exhausted the metabolites bind to hepatic macromolecules resulting in hepatic damage. N-acetylcystine can reduce the binding of electrophilic metabolite to hepatic proteins. The result of covalent binding of metabolites to tissue proteins can be direct cytotoxicity or initiation of an immunogenic response.

12.3.2.1 Immunogenic abnormal response : Drugs may stimulate antibody production because of their molecular character and cause tissue injury. The antibody so formed can attack the drug attached to a cell by covalent linkage and destroy the cell as in pinicillin induced hemolytic anemia. Another example is quinidine induced thrombocytopenia. Here drug induced antibody antigen complex is absorbed by the cell which is destroyed by activation of complement. Hydralazine and procainamide can chemically alter nuclear material that can stimulate formation of antinuclear antibody and may cause lupus erythematosus. Drug induced red cell aplasia can also arise out of immunologic reactions. It has been shown that red cell formation in bone marrow can be inhibited by phenytoin through immunologic reactions. Stimulation of antibody formation or sensitization of lymphocytes by a drug or one of its metabolites requires activation and covalent linkage to a protein or nucleic acid forms the basis for such toxicity.

Penicillin is well known for causing serum sickness because of deposition of circulating drug antibody complex on endothelial cell surface of tissues, which releases histamine that can produce hypotension characteristic of anaphylaxis, urticaria or wheezing and rhinorrhea.

Drugs may excite cell mediated immune response in case of topically administered agents which reacts with amino group or sulfhydril groups in the skin tissue and then with sensitized lymphocytes to produce skin rash (contact dermatitis).

12.3.2.3 Disturbances in the metabolic function of drugs : Drug toxicity can be associated with enzymatic defects such as deficiency of glucose-6-phosphate dehydrogenase (g6PD) can induce hemolytic anemia with a number of drugs such as primaquine, dapsone, nalidixic acid, nitrofurantoin and probenecid. The other drug toxicity associated with enzymatic defects are encountered in different porphyrias which may be erythropoietic or of hepatic origin acquired by disturbances in heme biosynthesis. Porphyrins are tetrapyrrole intermediates formed from delta-amino levulinic acid and porphobilinogen, the ferrous ion complex of porphobilinogen (heme) serves as prosthetic group for hemoprotein like hemoglobin. Porphyrias are characterized by overproduction, accumulation and excretion of intermediates of heme biosynthesis. Porphyria is life theratening and is precipitated by a variety of drugs, hormones and other agents. Porphyria exacerbation can be shown by barbiturates chlordiazepoxide, chlorpropamide, estrogen, griseofulvin, phenytoin and rifampin. During an acute attack there is increased urinary excretion of delta-amino levulinic acid and porphobilinogen.

12.4. MISCELLANEOUS DRUG EFFECTS

12.4.1. Drug Allergy

Drug allergy is the specific hypersensitiveness shown by individuals to a particular drug, which can be manifested in the form of skin eruption, eosinophilia, odema or anaphylactoid reactions and shock resulting from release of histamine, 5HT or other vasoactive substances. The machanism of drug allergy can be explained on the basis of immunological reactions. It has been shown that a class of immunoglobulins (IgE) takes part in the sensitization reaction of the tissue to any allergen. In this process blood basophils and tissue mast cells are activated to release the vasoactive substances and giving rise to hypersensitivity reactions.

Four types of hypersensitivity reactions are generally associated with drug induced allergic reaction.

(a) IgE class of immunoglobulins mediated allergic reactions: These give rise to urticaria, bronchospasm.

(b) IgG or IgM class of immunoglobulins are involved in allergic reactions that are complement dependent. In this the antibody is fixed to a circulating blood cell subject to a complement dependent lysis.

This results into an *autoimmune syndrome*, e.g. the phenomenon of lupus erythematosus following hydralazine therapy. The other examples are hemolytic anemia resulting from methyl dopa administration or thrombocytopenia due to quinidine and agranulocytosis due to number of other drugs which can be explained on the basis of autoimmune reactions. These reactions generally subside after the drug is withdrawn.

(c) *Serum sickness* to a drug are associated with IgG imunoglobulins, in which arthralgia, lymphadenopathy and drug fever may occur. These reactions generally last for 6 to 12 days and subside only after the drug is eliminated from the body. Corticosteroids are indicated to treat serum sickness.

(d) *Contact dermatitis* is cell mediated allergy arising out of topical application of a drug.

12.4.2 Drug Tolerance

Individuals have been found to be refractory to some drugs and chemical agents which normally will produce all the specified pharmacological effects on any other individual. The term tolerance can be defind as an exihibition of unusual resistance to all normal therapeutic as well as the toxic effects of a drug. It has been observed that rabbits are capable of enduring the unfavourable effects of atropine, this is reffered as species tolerance. Also it is reported that ephedrine is a poor mydriatic in some African nationals.

Tolerance can be acquired by repeated administration of the drug over a long period. This can be seen in opium and nicotine addicts. Drug tolerance can be attributed to icreased rate of excretion or the tissue cells may acquire the power to catabolize the drug. Pathogenic organisms may acquire tolerance through different mechanisms. Bacteria can adapt different metabolic path ways in its growth process giving rise to resistant orgnisms, most common example being the formationof sulpha drug and streptomycin resistant organisms.

12.4.3. Drug Resistance

Drug resistance can be of genetic or non genetic origin. In treatment of mcrobial infections we encounter some micro organisms that can survive in the host tissue for many years after the infection and are restrained by the host's defence mechanisms and so do not multiply. Such organisms are drug resistant and can not be eradicated. This type of drug resistance is of nongenetic origin. The examples of such infections are tuberculosis and leprosy. However if such organisms start proliferating then their offsprings will be fully susceptible to the same group of drugs which were earlier ineffective to eradicate. The other form of non genetic drug resistance can be because the microorganisms may lose the specific target structure on which the drugs act for its destruction. As for example penicillin susceptible organisms change their forms of protoplast during the course of penicillin treatment with the formation of organisms lacking cell wall so they become resistant to cell wall inhibitor drugs like cephalosporins or penicillins.

Drug Resistance of Genetic Origin

Pathogenic microbes have emerged as a result of genetic changes and subsequent selection processes. Such changes can be chromosomal or extra chromosomal. Bacterial chromosomes are made of double stranded DNA molecules which guide the further replication process of the bacteria in an orderly manner. Drug resistance can develop out of chromosomal factors because in the presence of drugs formation of chromosomal mutants can occur spontaneously. For example the formation of chromosomal mutants to antitubercular drug like rifampin occurs very fast, so treatment of an infection with rifampin as a sole drug fails.

Extra chromosomal bacterial resistance to a drug can occur because of aberration in the genetic material known as plasmids. Plasmid are circular DNA molecules that reproduce themselves and are thus conserved, apart from the chromosome, through successive cell division. Plasmids control the formation of enzymes capable of destroying anti-microbial drugs. For example plasmid determine resistance to penicillins and cyclosporins by carrying genes for the formation of beta lactamases. Lastly microorganisms acquire resistance to drugs because they share a common mechanism of action. Such drug resistance is reffered as the process of cross resistance.

12.4.4 Drug Abuse

Misuse of chemicals and drugs for nonmedical purposes can be termed as drug abuse. WHO has defined drug abuse as "persistent or sporadic use inconsistant with or unrelated to acceptable medical practice. The following group of agents and drugs are generally put to misuse which lead to development of dependence both psychic and physical leading to addiction.

(a) **Hallucinogens :** Cannabis, hashish, marihuana and heroin. None of these agents are therapeutically used for any purpose. They are potent hallucinogens and are mostly used by drug abusers for their optical and acoustic hallucinating actions. These agents induce a sense of perception such as sight, touch, sound, smell or taste that has no basis in external stimulation.

(b) **Hypnotics sedatives and Opioids :** These groups of drugs initially may be used for a specific therapeutic purpose. However they have the capacity to induce physical dependence as for example morphine, pentazocine, phenobarbital and many others. If these group of durgs are used for a long period and then withdrawn they may induce tremor, profuse sweating, restlessness, lacrimation, uncontrolable yawning, stomach pain and muscle aching. These are few of the signs of drug dependence.

(c) **Stimulants :** Amphetamine and phenmetrazine are the stimulant group of drugs that induce drug dependence. Amphetamine has very limited theraeutic use, however amphetamine preparations like Dexedrine (dexamphetamine), Methedrine (methyl amphetamine) are widely misused. Methedrine can be manufactured from ephedrine. All amphetamine users take the drug for its psychic effect. In low dose they feel energetic, and do not feel the need of sleep or food. However they are prone to excessive mood swings, particularly while withdrawing from the drug.

Tolerance to the mental effect of all drugs of misuse develops with chronic use and there is a need for ever increasing amounts to sustain the desired euphoriant effect which loads to morbidity.

Curiosity and social pressure are the strongest factors in drug misuse.

INDEX

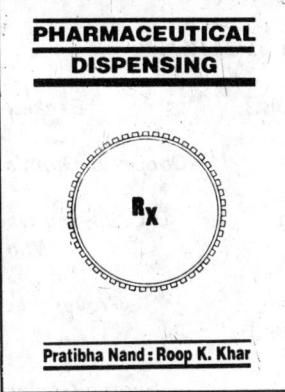
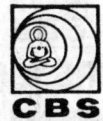

CBS OUTSTANDING BOOKS

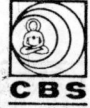

CBS

CBS PUBLISHERS & DISTRIBUTORS

4596/1-A, 11 Daryaganj, New Delhi-110002 (India)